IT'S
PROBABLY
NOTHING

IT'S PROBABLY NOTHING

The Stress-Less Guide to Dealing with Health Anxiety, Wellness Fads, and Overhyped Headlines

CASEY GUEREN

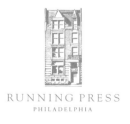

Running Press

PHILADELPHIA

Copyright © 2021 by Casey Gueren
Cover copyright © 2021 by Hachette Book Group, Inc.
Foreword copyright © 2021 by Dr. Jen Gunter

Running Press
Hachette Book Group
1290 Avenue of the Americas, New York, NY 10104
www.runningpress.com
@Running_Press

Printed in China

First Edition: September 2021

Published by Running Press, an imprint of Perseus Books, LLC, a subsidiary of Hachette Book Group, Inc. The Running Press name and logo is a trademark of the Hachette Book Group.

The Hachette Speakers Bureau provides a wide range of authors for speaking events. To find out more, go to www.hachettespeakersbureau.com or call (866) 376-6591.

The publisher is not responsible for websites (or their content) that are not owned by the publisher.

Print book cover and interior design by Susan Van Horn.

Library of Congress Control Number: 2021936382

ISBNs: 978-0-7624-7183-6 (paperback), 978-0-7624-7182-9 (ebook)

RRD-S

10 9 8 7 6 5 4 3 2 1

CONTENTS

FOREWORD

HAVE YOU EVER GOOGLED YOUR MEDICAL SYMPTOMS IN THE middle of the night?

It should come as no surprise to learn you're not alone. Almost everyone has researched health information online, either for themselves or a loved one, or both. I know that my own patients do it, and at times I know they feel guilty when they tell me, although they shouldn't. Having access to quality information online shouldn't just be the privilege of the few in medicine—it is everyone's right.

It's not uncommon for me to encounter one of my patients who has spent hours online—maybe even longer—looking up symptoms, researching a diagnosis, or investigating therapies. This excites me because it means my patient is engaged and wants to learn more about their health. The downside is the information they have gathered is often incorrect. It may be alarmist, recommend unnecessary tests, or be the gateway to a snake oil-fest of epic proportions.

It isn't their fault. When you research health information online using standard internet search techniques what happens is a popularity contest: search engines favor quantity or number of previous clicks over quality of the content. And with companies (both pharmaceutical and those making supplements) and influencers affecting the results, the algorithm seems to favor everyone and everything . . . with the exception of unbiased, factual information. What typically makes these searches even less effective is that they often happen late at night, which is not the ideal time to conduct health research—especially your own. It seems the odds of coming away less informed or misinformed from your search are at least as high (if not higher) than coming away better educated about your health.

The internet can be the most amazing medical library out there, and it can also literally be the worst, but even the best library is of little value if you don't know how to use it. Search for "cervical cancer prevention" online and you might end up on a guide to getting the HPV vaccine (yeah!) and how to advocate for getting the vaccine if your doctor dismisses your request (practical and helpful!). Or you might stumble upon a wellness influencer with over 100,000 followers on Instagram who claims that Pap smears are unnecessary because "you know your body" and hence can detect if there is a problem (an ignorant and dangerous position that could kill people with a cervix—and yes, this is a real example).

It shouldn't be this kind of crap shoot.

But it's not just because basic health education in our schools is lacking, and most people don't ever learn how to look for medical information online. I probably don't need to tell you that good content is often inaccessible (and, let's face it, sometimes snooze-worthy), while wellness fads rule on social media. It's not surprising that the health and wellness corner of the internet is a quagmire.

Casey Gueren knows this all too well. She is a writer and health editor (who I have had the pleasure of writing for) and she's not afraid to admit that she is often very anxious about her health. So she gets it. Really. Not just the worries that many of us (doctors included) have when we search for health information online, but also the importance of learning how to access that information—because, in many cases, she put it there. What makes this book unique is Casey's insight into the creation of online health information. She spent years writing the types of headlines that will catch your eye and the content you might find yourself reading in the middle of the night. She has also covered the wellness industry and health fads as both a journalist and a curious consumer. She's been there.

She's not going to tell you to stay off the internet, but she will help you navigate it in a way that's less stressful and more helpful. With the right tools, the internet is an amazing medical library that can help people learn more about their health and how to advocate for the best care. With the wrong set of directions, the internet is a fast track to misinformation, misdiagnoses, and even medical conspiracy theories. It can stoke our fear and lead to over-testing or splurging on unnecessary and potentially harmful supplements.

In this book Casey becomes that virtual best friend you text in the middle of the night with a random health question—but one who understands the concerns that send you online and how to separate the medical from the mystical when you are staring at your screen. Casey gives her readers an essential toolkit for navigating medical information online in the age of clickbait stories and shady wellness schemes.

This is an accessible, funny, relevant, and at times poignant guide to online health literacy from someone who has been behind the scenes creating content and is ready to share her backstage pass with you.

Jen Gunter, MD
@DrJenGunter

INTRODUCTION

NO, IT'S NOT JUST YOU.

YOU KNOW WHAT'S EVEN MORE FRUSTRATING THAN GOOGLING your symptoms on a Friday night, convinced that you're dying?

Googling your symptoms on a Friday night and landing on an article that *you* wrote on the topic. And—despite the nice, reassuring tone—still not believing that you're not dying.

Yeah, I've done that.

A few years ago, I was about to head out to a party when my gynecologist called. Now, as a health editor, I'd written enough articles about vaginas to know that your gynecologist usually doesn't call at 5 p.m. on a Friday night with news that everything is cool. I could hear my heartbeat in my ears as she explained that she had found atypical cells in my latest Pap smear. "It could be nothing," she said, "but we'll want you to come back in for a biopsy soon."

I ripped off my jacket, suddenly feeling hot and sick. Then came the classic tunnel vision, chest pain, and numbness that anyone who has experienced a panic attack might be familiar with.

At that moment, it didn't matter that I was an award-winning health journalist. It didn't matter that I had written several different articles about Pap smears and everything that can cause a wonky result. My mind ignored all of the rational, reasonable information I had heard and written over the years and immediately bounced between possibilities like sexually transmitted infections, infertility, cancer, and death.

I started searching around online—even though I knew better—and within minutes I was on an article that *I* had written a few years prior. "Don't panic," I wrote in 2015.

Psh . . . what does she know, I thought.

I continued down this internet rabbit hole for about 10 minutes, searching for something that didn't exist: an authority that would tell me with certainty that everything was going to be okay. Instead, my eyes darted to every worst-case scenario on every page, latching on to any sentence that started with "In rare cases . . ."

Eventually I closed the laptop and the panic slowly subsided, receding enough for me to leave the apartment. But that anxiety stayed with me for weeks, until the biopsy came back: normal.

This was not the first or the last time my health anxiety sent me into a panic. To be honest, I can't remember a time when I didn't scrutinize every mark, bump, or feeling, wondering if it was "normal" . . . then assuming that it wasn't. A lump on my head was a tumor. A pounding headache was cancer. A racing heart was clearly something fatal and definitely not a reasonable side effect of the giant cold brew I had just downed.

And yet, in spite of—or maybe because of—my ever-present health anxiety, I've spent the bulk of my career as a health writer and editor for some pretty popular media brands: *Cosmopolitan, Women's Health,* BuzzFeed, *SELF.*

That's right, this health journalist is also quite the *hypochondriac.*[*] It's

---

[*]Heads up: *Hypochondriac* is an outdated term that I'm using here for familiarity's sake. I'll explain more about the loaded connotations of this term—and what you can use instead—later on in this section.

exhausting. Or, it *was* exhausting—so exhausting in fact that, in the span of writing this book, I quit my job. But more on that later.

• • • • • • • • • • • • • • • • • • •

I've always been a little too preoccupied with my body. Maybe you can relate. One of many early memories of this comes to mind: I was a teenager casually riding in the car with my mom and went from zero to oh-my-god-I-have-cancer in record time.

"There's a lump on my head."

I was in the front passenger seat of my mom's car, my elbow resting on the door and my hand cradling the side of my face, when my finger grazed against something under my hair that was slightly raised.

"It's probably nothing," my mom said.

But it felt like something.

Actually, I can't remember exactly what it felt like—I must have been 15 or 16 at the time—but I vividly remember the sensation that something was wrong. I spent the rest of the drive subtly surveying the surface of my skull, my fingers blindly feeling around under my hair. *Did I have the same bump on the other side of my head? That would make it less suspicious. Did it hurt? If it hurt, it probably wasn't cancer—I think I read that somewhere.*

It could have been a zit, a clogged hair follicle, or literally just what my head felt like, but at the time, I was filled with this overwhelming certainty that it was something awful.

My poor mom. She was used to my random body worries at that point and probably just tried her best not to engage. I would usually forget about it soon enough—often around the time I was distracted from whatever symptom I was currently obsessing over: a headache, a weird pain, a mole I never noticed before, a stomachache, a suspicious heartbeat, whatever.

This preoccupation with my health started well before WebMD and Google made wondering "Am I dying?" basically a hobby. Clickbait articles might not have existed yet, but there were plenty of terrifying health stories in women's magazines to satisfy my imagination and anxiety. I remember thinking that toxic shock syndrome was definitely going to take me out one day—but not before I got herpes, ovarian cancer, and an ectopic pregnancy. My body was, in all likelihood, a ticking time bomb.

My mom probably figured that her anxious little girl was going through a weird phase and would eventually stop assuming that all her headaches were brain tumors.

Reader: She did not.

Instead, she grew up to become a health editor, covering every ailment you could possibly imagine and a few you've probably never heard of.

Was this a healthy coping mechanism or a very poor career choice? Hard to say! But it's given me a lot of insight into how the messages we're getting every day can impact the way we think about our health, the way we take care of our bodies, and the way we react when something feels off.

And it's also helped me realize that I'm not the only one who is completely unsatisfied with the response, "It's probably nothing." Whether it's coming from your doctor, your mom, your best friend, or your computer screen, this simple phrase can be so damn frustrating, even when it's filled with the best of intentions. It's a phrase that suggests reassurance while at the same time admitting uncertainty.

And, hey, I say it all the time, too. I say it to myself (a lot!) when I'm trying to downplay my latest health concern. I say it to my friend when he's freaking out about a rash that is most likely razor burn—not bedbugs. I say it in an article when writing about an often-searched symptom that is *almost always* no big deal.

But when most of us hear, "It's probably nothing," our reaction is usually, "Okay, but it *could* be something."

And if that resonates with you—hi, you're my people. This book is for you! If you've also panicked about a weird symptom, Googled your health concerns, fallen for wellness fads on social media, and struggled to know where to turn, which source to believe, or what to do to take care of yourself . . . you're not alone. I can definitely relate. I can also help.

· · · · · · · · · · · · · · · · · · ·

You might be wondering at this point why you should listen to me. That's fair—I clearly have a hard time taking my own advice occasionally, too. But as someone who has worked in the wellness industry for close to a decade— where I've had a seat at the table next to public health experts, medical professionals, health journalists, and wellness entrepreneurs—I picked up on a few things I think are worth sharing:

1. Most of us have a lot of questions and concerns about our bodies and our health. Trust me, I've seen what you Google. It's not just you.

2. There are significant barriers when it comes to accessing quality, affordable, empathetic health care. So it's no wonder we spend so much time, money, and energy looking for fast fixes. It's no wonder we fall victim to predatory wellness practices that lack science but lead with empathy.

3. It is really freaking hard to navigate the barrage of health information and misinformation being hurled at us from all angles. It can feel impossible to know who to trust, what to believe, and how to actually take care of yourself.

Here's the thing: I can't cure your health anxiety, fix the health care system, or banish health misinformation. That's not what you'll find in this book. But what I can do from my corner of the wellness industry is help you navigate all of that a bit more easily. I can help you feel less alone when you're stressed out about your body. I can boost your health literacy as well as your wellness bullshit detector. I can give you the tools to better understand and act on the latest health news. Hopefully, I can make this whole unnecessarily complicated process of finding answers to your health questions suck just a little bit less.

That's because I've been on both sides of the search engine—panicking about my own problems while also writing and editing so much of the health content that you end up clicking on in a panic. I know how frustrating all of this is, and I think—I hope—my experience can help.

So, if that all sounds good to you, let me tell you a bit more about who I am and how I got here . . .

· · · · · · · · · · · · · · · · · · ·

My career in health writing started not-so-innocently enough. My first job out of college was at *Cosmopolitan* magazine as an editorial assistant, and I was eager to write about anything and everything. And, obviously, the health articles especially piqued my interest, because those were always the first pages I read when I got the magazine as a teenager.

Of course, I didn't mention to my coworkers that the health section was also what brought me the most anxiety as a teenager. They didn't need to know that.

During my early days, one of the editors at the magazine needed help with a story. There was a rumor going around that "semen facials" were a thing being offered at actual spas, and the editor wanted to write about what benefits, theoretically, might come from putting cum on your face. (So, yes, if you're wondering, working at *Cosmo* in the 2000s was exactly like you think it was.) The editor asked me to try to find a dermatologist to talk to me about it. Overeager, 22-year-old me took this assignment *very* seriously.

I made a lot of cold calls and left a lot of voicemails before realizing that everyone definitely thought I was prank calling them. Eventually, a real live board-certified dermatologist based out of Miami called me back. She talked to me about the proteins that might live in sperm and how some proteins are technically beneficial in skin care. So basically, it's a thing you *can* put on your face, but don't expect to swap it for your nightly retinol and see miraculous benefits.

I know it sounds like a silly assignment, but it felt like *journalism.* I ran my interview notes over to the editor. She seemed thrilled and honestly impressed that I had gotten anyone to answer the phone, let alone talk to me about sperm facials. I don't think the story ever ended up running. But it didn't matter, I felt like a reporter. And that's how I got into health writing.

Looking back on it now, health reporting was a natural fit for someone who always had an endless loop of health and body questions running through her head. My editors praised me for always offering up so many creative but relatable pitches, when in reality I was just mining my own anxieties:

○ **12 Things That Can Cause Boob Pain**

○ **How Pregnant Can This Get You?**

○ **How to Tell If It's an Ingrown Hair or Herpes**

Soon enough, they let me write the two recurring health pages in *Cosmo* every month. Over the next handful of years, I would go from those two little health pages to becoming a senior digital editor at *Women's Health* magazine, to overseeing the entire health section at BuzzFeed, to eventually being hired as health director at *SELF* magazine.

I had found my niche. I made a career out of finding answers to my own—and everyone else's—health questions. It was interesting, rewarding, and almost never boring, because we all have questions and anxieties when it comes to our bodies and our health.

Some of us just have more than others.

• • • • • • • • • • • • • • • • • • •

Most people who worked with me or read my articles probably never realized that I was just as scared, stressed, and confused about my health as they were about theirs. Probably more so, to be honest. Despite my years of health reporting and access to some of the best medical experts out there, I still occasionally panic and dive down the same ridiculous search holes that you do. I still read a list of possible reasons why I'm tired and think, *yep, cancer.* I still attribute a random tremor to something fatal, instead of the most likely culprit: the excessive amounts of caffeine I'm drinking.

So, real talk time: I've spent nearly a decade as a health writer and editor, but I've spent much longer than that being very anxious about my own health. I've been convinced I had a brain tumor, a blood clot, a heart attack, anaphylaxis, diabetes, an ectopic pregnancy, a regular pregnancy—you know, all the usual suspects.

I had, of course, heard the term *hypochondriac* before. But I definitely didn't see myself or my concerns that way. I associated that term with people who were constantly going to doctors and refusing to leave without a diagnosis. I was on the opposite end of the spectrum: privately panicking about something I was sure was killing me, while avoiding an annual checkup I assumed would just confirm my worst fears. *I'm not being a hypochondriac,* I thought. *Those people are delusional—I'm the person you read about that was young and healthy before she developed a rare rodent-borne virus and never recovered. YOU'LL SEE.*

I still didn't know that this near-constant anxiety I was dealing with had a name. But I knew that I was avoiding things that might trigger it. Once, while reading a magazine on a plane, I flipped right past an article about a young woman whose ambiguous symptoms turned out to be cancer. *Nope, not for me, will definitely think I have that.*

And yes, unfortunately, this meant avoiding things at work, too. My job was inherently triggering for me at times. While covering a big editorial package around type 2 diabetes, I became more and more convinced that I had it with every article I wrote or edited. At one point, I barely skimmed a feature

I was supposed to be editing, afraid that the more information I picked up in the story, the more it would confirm the anxious thoughts already swirling in my head. (Luckily I had some amazing writers and editors working for me, so the articles were fine, I promise!)

I avoided doctor's appointments, too. I was a health editor who was skipping her annual physicals while constantly ending my own articles with some variation of: "If you're ever concerned, check in with your primary care provider." (Meanwhile, urgent care was basically my primary care provider.)

But most of all, I avoided telling anyone what was really going on inside my head. Right now, in this book, is the first time I've ever spoken publicly about this.

The difference between "being a hypochondriac" and having health anxiety

The term *hypochondriac* gets thrown around a lot. "I'm such a hypochondriac!" you might say when you're convinced you're getting sick, when you're worried that your thinning hair must be a sign of a hormonal disorder, or literally anytime you watch *Grey's Anatomy* and happen to have one of the symptoms the terminal patient has.

But what you may not know is that "being a hypochondriac" isn't actually a clinically recognized disorder anymore. The term fell out of favor in the last decade for a few reasons. For starters, the term *hypochondriac* was seen as pretty pejorative and stigmatizing. But it was also too broad in scope for the variety of ways people can experience anxiety around their health.

The last time hypochondriasis was classified as a mental health condition was back before 2013, in the fourth edition of the Diagnostic and Statistical Manual of Mental Disorders (DSM-IV). The DSM is basically the go-to resource for mental health professionals to diagnose and treat conditions, developed by the American Psychiatric Association. This manual is what determines what constitutes a mental health condition, how it's diagnosed, how it's treated—all that good stuff. In the DSM-IV, *hypochondriasis* was used to describe someone who is preoccupied with the idea that they have a serious disease—or the fear around having a disease—based on some kind of misinterpretation of their symptoms, and these concerns don't go away, regardless of medical attention or reassurance.

Then things changed with the fifth edition of the DSM (known as the DSM-5), which was published in 2013. In that edition, hypochondriasis was axed from the manual and replaced with two mental health conditions: somatic symptom disorder and illness anxiety disorder. Both of these diagnoses still center around severe and persistent symptoms of health anxiety, like what many of us think of when we think about *hypochondriasis*. The difference between the two is that somatic symptom disorder is characterized by a preoccupation with *specific* physical symptoms, while illness anxiety disorder is characterized by ongoing health anxiety even *without* physical symptoms.

This may all just seem like semantics—who cares what something is called, really? Well, it matters to researchers and mental health professionals who can better study, diagnose, and treat a condition when it's clearly defined. And it matters to the person who has been dealing with these symptoms for a long time, never knowing that the underlying condition had a name—or a treatment. Hell, I was a health editor and even I didn't know.

Remember—I didn't consider myself a *hypochondriac*. But when I started reading about illness anxiety disorder . . . wow, it was like reading your horoscope and feeling some mixture of seen and personally attacked by the accuracy. It perfectly described the thoughts and behaviors I'd had for so long.

According to the DSM-5, here are the criteria for being diagnosed with illness anxiety disorder:[1]

- Preoccupation with having or acquiring a serious illness.

- Somatic symptoms are not present or, if present, are only mild in intensity. If another medical condition is present or there is a high risk for developing a medical condition (e.g., strong family history is present), the preoccupation is clearly excessive or disproportionate. There is a high level of anxiety about health, and the individual is easily alarmed about personal health status.

- The individual performs excessive health-related behaviors (e.g., repeatedly checks his or her body for signs of illness) or exhibits maladaptive avoidance (e.g., avoids doctor appointments and hospitals).

- Illness preoccupation has been present for at least six months, but the specific illness that is feared may change over that period of time.

- The illness-related preoccupation is not better explained by another mental disorder, such as somatic symptom disorder, panic disorder, generalized anxiety disorder, body dysmorphic disorder, obsessive-compulsive disorder, or delusional disorder, somatic type.

Source: DSM-5

Hi, hello, that is me.

As someone who had a pretty limited understanding of hypochondriasis my whole life, I get why the American Psychiatric Association narrowed the focus. But what really got my attention was this note at the bottom of the criteria for illness anxiety disorder:

Specify whether:

CARE-SEEKING TYPE: Medical care, including physician visits or undergoing tests and procedures, is frequently used.

CARE-AVOIDANT TYPE: Medical care is rarely used.

Source: DSM-5

Welp, there it is. People might associate "being a hypochondriac" with hopping from doctor to doctor, desperate for a diagnosis, but that's not how health anxiety manifests for everyone.

Jonathan S. Abramowitz, PhD, professor of psychology and neuroscience at the University of North Carolina at Chapel Hill and editor-in-chief of the *Journal of Obsessive-Compulsive and Related Disorders*, explained to me the evolution of the condition over the past few decades. The change in the DSM, he says, reflects a shift in the understanding of what might be behind these thoughts and behaviors.

"Instead of people thinking that hypochondriacs just wanted all this attention from doctors, people started to look into—wait a minute, these are folks that have legitimate worries about their bodies, about illnesses. They're not making this stuff up. They're noticing body sensations that they're worried about," explains Abramowitz. "The body sensations don't indicate that there's something wrong, but they're noticing something, and they're responding to that. And they have catastrophic fears and beliefs, just like people with other problems with anxiety, like panic, OCD, stuff like that."

Obviously not everyone experiences the same level of health anxiety I do, but most people can relate to being "a bit of a hypochondriac," at least some of the time. "It's really common," says Abramowitz. "Because, after all, our health is the most important thing, so it's certainly something that it's easy for people to get anxious about. We pay a lot of attention to our bodies because we're in our bodies. It's easy to say, 'Oh no, what was that?'"

So much of mental health exists on a spectrum. You can be anxious without having generalized anxiety disorder. You can feel depressed without having major depression. You can have intrusive thoughts or compulsive behaviors without having obsessive-compulsive disorder. And you can experience health anxiety without meeting the specific criteria for illness anxiety disorder or somatic symptom disorder.

It's hard to say for sure how many people experience health anxiety, mainly because we barely know how many people meet the criteria for these actual diagnoses. The DSM-5 estimates that anywhere from 1.3 to 10 percent of adults in the U.S. have illness anxiety disorder, while 5 to 7 percent of adults have somatic symptom disorder.[2] But many experts aren't too keen on those estimates.

"We don't have very good estimates, and the reason is folks don't often go to psychologists. They go to physicians," says Abramowitz.

It makes sense. When you're anxious about your health, you don't go to a therapist; you go to the doctor—or, more likely, Dr. Google. Sure, some people may eventually end up in front of a mental health professional who diagnoses them with a clinical form of health anxiety, but many don't.

Plus, this doesn't account for all those people who experience health anxiety on an occasional basis—like being convinced you have a blood clot after a long flight, or being paranoid about the latest outbreak all over the news, or wondering if that weird head pain is more than just a headache. If you picked up this book, I'm willing to bet you can relate to this.

Heads up: the wellness industry knows you're not okay.

What I've learned from nearly a decade covering health and wellness is this: Everyone is a little bit scared, confused, and stressed out about their bodies. And I'm hardly the first one to figure this out.

It's no coincidence that more and more companies are bombarding women with the message that they need to pay money to fix imaginary problems with their bodies (think: vaginal odor, cellulite, occasional gas and bloating, not having an orgasm in five minutes—you get the point). Despite—or maybe because of—the significant barriers to accessing health care, the wellness industry is out there *thriving*.

The global wellness economy was reported to be a $4.5 trillion market in 2018, according to a report by the Global Wellness Institute.[3] And that doesn't shock me. Over the past decade, I've watched as many people have felt ignored by their doctors, sidelined by our health care system, and eager to take a larger role in their own health. The booming wellness industry answered that call-to-action, and pretty soon we were up to our ears in CBD oil and health trackers.

There are undoubtedly positive effects of health tech, wellness startups, and health industry disruptors, but there are also companies out there cashing in on this culture shift by peddling snake oil for whatever you're currently stressing about. At best, these things are a waste of money—like most supplements and CBD lattes—but at worst, they could actually be harmful—like "detoxing" your vagina with douches, which could increase your risk of pelvic inflammatory disease.

My job as a health editor was to help readers make sense of it all. Now, I want to give you the tools to be more informed and less freaked out when it comes to your own body. I want to help boost your health literacy, your media literacy, and your wellness bullshit detector. I've been the gatekeeper long enough. Now, I'm propping the door open and inviting you in.

This book is for everyone who needs a little help separating hype from health. And right now, that's pretty much all of us.

When I made the decision in 2020 to leave my job as a full-time health editor in the middle of a pandemic, it wasn't easy. In fact, I would argue that there had never been a time when more people depended on the media for health information than in 2020. How could I walk away from that? As a health editor with health anxiety, living through and reporting on a literal pandemic was basically my moment, right?

Yeah, it was. And that was one hard-ass moment. It felt like the instant when a wave pushes you under the water and you're knocked around so much you don't even know which way is up. And I was one of the fortunate ones.

At that point, I had already signed on to write this book. I was spending longer-than-ever days making sure *SELF* was reporting on COVID-19 from every responsible angle, and I was also spending my mornings, nights, and weekends trying to write a book about how to tame your health anxiety and navigate the minefield of health misinformation and wellness hype that contribute to it. Juggling this workload while living in the epicenter of the pandemic and dealing with my own anxious body thoughts every single day was no easy task.

It's no coincidence that in the span of writing this book I quit my job in health media. Drilling up all of this self-reflection and behind-the-scenes insight was draining, to say the least. Not to mention my 9-to-5 (ha, who are we kidding, 9-to-7? Sometimes 9?) was spent managing health lineups and health reporters through a truly unmanageable time. I needed a break. I needed distance. I needed to play to my strengths in a time when everyone's capacity was at it's absolute lowest. I needed to ask myself how and where I could be most helpful.

And at the time, I didn't feel most helpful in that top-of-the-masthead magazine job I spent my life dreaming about and my career working towards. When I envisioned this moment as a teenager pouring over a stack of magazines, I imagined fewer panic attacks. Maybe not zero panic attacks, just fewer.

But in those mornings, nights, and weekends when I wrote this book—when I wrote about how to decode and debunk the health headlines, how to challenge your anxious health thoughts, and how to boost your health literacy—that's when I felt like I was onto something. Maybe I could jump off the media ladder I had been climbing ever since I could remember and still make an impact from the sidelines.

So I quit my job as an executive editor and buckled down on this book: my health media manifesto filled with a whole lot of insights only a long-time health editor with health anxiety can really tell you.

Here's what you're going to learn in this book.

I often wonder what it would be like if everyone had the same health literacy tools I've gained from my time as a health journalist—whether it's about knowing how to interpret those scary vaping headlines or figuring out if celery juice is actually a miracle cure or even just wondering what that itch is. This book will give you the same tools and tricks that I used both in covering complicated health topics and in troubleshooting personal health problems. As someone who's experienced health anxiety for most of my life, I've found that the tools that helped me be a better editor also allowed me to navigate my own health issues more calmly and effectively.

Don't worry, I'm not going to tell you to never Google a health question again. In fact, go ahead—you'll probably land on an article I wrote or edited, and hopefully it'll be helpful in alleviating your concerns. But I can do you one better: What if I could give you the same tactics I used as a journalist to boost your own health literacy? If they worked for someone like me—someone who spent most of her life convinced her body was a ticking time bomb—they can probably help you, too.

In Part I, I'm going to cover:

- Why we're so starved for health information

- Why looking up our symptoms online is so damn tempting, but also ultimately adding to our anxiety

- How the wellness industry is fueled by and contributing to our stress

I'm covering those basics first, because understanding *why* you stress about your health is so crucial to doing something about it. It gives you the framework to start noticing and challenging the thoughts and behaviors that are keeping you trapped in that cycle.

Then, in Part II, you're going to learn the tools and tricks to boost your health literacy, your wellness bullshit detector, and your care toolkit. You're going to find out:

- How to listen to your body . . . just enough

- How to not freak out over every health headline you read

- How to not fall for the latest wellness trend all over Instagram

- How to tackle a health question like a health editor

- How to get the inclusive, empathetic, evidence-based care you deserve

So take a deep breath, grab a cup of something soothing—coffee, tea, wine, whatever—and let's get started.

A NOTE ABOUT "NORMAL"

Before I get too far, I want to have a chat about the word *normal*, because it's a word we hear and say a lot when talking about our bodies and our health. Most of the health articles I wrote and edited throughout my career were in response to that nagging question so many of us have had at one point: Is this thing on or in my body "normal"? Am *I* "normal"?

It took a lot of reporting, self-reflection, and complicated discussions with experts and colleagues over the years to help me understand why we keep coming back to this question—and why it's such a flawed question to begin with.

You should know that there is nothing wrong with you for asking. After all, we're constantly bombarded with the message that there's something wrong with our bodies. *You're not sleeping enough or you're sleeping too much. You're eating too much meat or not getting enough protein. Something on your body shouldn't look, feel, or smell like that.*

No wonder we're so preoccupied with what's "normal."

But it's important to recognize that our obsession with having a "normal" body is deeply rooted in ableism. While it may be common and conversational to throw around the word *normal* when we're talking about bodies and health, that kind of language perpetuates the pervasive belief that there is a right and a wrong way to have a body. And I realize this is a hard thing to unlearn, because pretty much every aspect of society *does* view certain bodies and states of health as "better" than others.

So let's get one thing straight: Your body is not abnormal if you have a chronic health condition or a disability. While there's no question that these can come with countless obstacles, that's because our society was built only to accommodate people whose bodies and health fit into a very narrow concept. Because of this—and the failings of our health care system—receiving a diagnosis of a chronic illness or disability can be terrifying.

But that diagnosis does not determine whether or not you are "normal." It doesn't define your value, your worth, your achievements, or your right to respect, decency, and agency. A diagnosis often tells you about the road ahead—and that road may be bumpy as fuck and paved with systems of marginalization that make it practically impossible to access quality care. It might be a very different road than the one you expected to be on. But it's the *road* that is broken and needs fixing. It's not you. Your body is normal, because all bodies are normal.

In this book, you'll notice that I put the word *normal* in quotation marks whenever I'm referring to that ingrained belief that there is a right and wrong way to have a body. And, whenever possible, I've tried to spell out exactly what I'm talking about instead—because many of us use "normal" to mean so many different things. Depending on the context, "normal" could be used to mean healthy, common, typical, harmless, or not worthy of concern. But "normal" can also be used to infer that anything more or less than that is abnormal, unnatural, undesirable, or otherwise subpar. And those descriptions should never be used to describe a person or a body.

Okay, glad we had this chat.

PART I

WHY WE CAN'T STOP STRESSING ABOUT OUR BODIES

T here were times while writing this book that I thought, *Does anyone really need this? Am I just writing this for me? Am I the only one who feels this way?*

But then something would happen to remind me just how not alone I am in wondering what the hell is wrong with my body or how in the world I'm supposed to be taking care of it.

○ Like getting a text from my friend frantically trying to figure out if she'd contracted flesh-eating bacteria from a recent dip in the Long Island Sound.

○ Or overhearing a conversation among highly informed colleagues about which cleanse is best for "a good detox."

○ Or seeing Facebook friends sharing "immune-boosting hacks" that had zero science behind them.

○ Or finding out that members of my own family didn't get the flu shot because they thought it could give you the flu.

None of those things are stupid or silly—they're reasonable reactions from reasonable people based on the information they have been given . . . or not given. The truth is, when it comes to figuring out how to take care of our bodies, we're all just doing our best with what we have—and unfortunately the information we have is kind of a clusterfuck most of the time.

So here's what I want you to keep in mind as you dive into this book: You have no reason to feel embarrassed or ashamed for having a whole lot of questions about your body and your health. But most of all, you should know you're definitely not the only one.

CHAPTER 1

Remember health class? Me neither.

THROUGHOUT MY CAREER, I'VE SPENT A LOT OF TIME ASKING A lot of doctors a lot of health questions:

- "What's up with that weird brown discharge?"

- "What can you tell me about nipple hair?"

- "How much peeing is too much peeing?"

- "What does it mean if you take a while to orgasm?"

- "Why would someone have this pain, this bump, this smell . . . ?"

And so often I get the same response from the medical experts: "That's normal."

It turns out, we are all really good at stressing out about typical body things that have a totally benign cause—like that you're tired or you're stressed or you're not drinking enough water. Sometimes all three for, like, weeks at a time, if we're being honest.

So why are we like this? Why is there such a chasm between what we probably *should* know about our bodies and what we *actually* know? Why are we so quick to panic about things that seem even remotely off? Listen, I've heard medical school is hard, so it's not like I expect us all to be experts on the human body, but you would think that we would have a better understanding of this bag of bones we're living in, right?

The truth is, many of us have just a basic understanding of our bodies and the way they work. As a result, it's common to misinterpret regular old bodily functions—or slight variations in those bodily functions—as something scary and serious.

I'm talking about things like:

- Headaches, exhaustion, nausea, brain fog, dizziness . . .

- Sweating, shivering, shaking, tingling, buzzing, throbbing, twitching, aching . . .

- Head pain, stomach pain, chest pain, boob pain, vagina pain, foot pain, side pain, back pain . . .

- Some "unusual" change in your sleep, your appetite, your bowel movements, your bladder, your period, your focus, your vision . . .

I'm willing to bet you've worried about several of those things, too. And why shouldn't you? As a former health editor, I'm well aware that all of those symptoms could be signs of something serious. But they can also just *happen* for tons of reasons that are not killing you.

I know what you're thinking (because I've thought it, too): "But what if that stomach pain *is* my appendix bursting? What if that chest pain *is* a heart attack? Isn't it better to be safe than sorry?" Of course, yes, if you think something is wrong, you should see a health care provider, always. The problem is, many of us don't actually do that. Getting to the doctor is a whole thing, and going to the hospital or urgent care can be even worse—especially if you don't have the time, money, insurance, transportation, childcare, and so on to do that. Most of the time, we turn to the internet instead.

I've analyzed enough search data to confirm that most of us Google the same body questions over and over. You may think your browser history is uniquely embarrassing, but I'm sure it's not. It's probably pretty average. In fact, let me just give you some numbers: In an average month, 282,000 people look up "vaginal itching," 134,000 people Google "breast pain," 120,000 people search "bloating meaning," and 25,400 type "period poop" into the search bar (if you know, you know).

> *You may think your browser history is uniquely embarrassing, but I'm sure it's not.*

Our bodies don't come with a user manual—though that would be dope. Many of us have a very basic understanding of the way bodies work, so it's no surprise that we're out here just trying our best to put the pieces together (like poop tending to get truly out of control around your period) and hoping that the internet will handle the rest. It's just so much easier and less awkward to ask your phone than it is to ask a real live medical professional.

When I worked at BuzzFeed, I used to host brainstorms where I asked people to come with the last question they had looked up about their body. (There was also an anonymous form they could fill out if they preferred.) The questions were weird and funny and ridiculous—but also completely valid! Things came up like:

○ **Does brown period blood mean I'm dying?**

○ **Why am I so sweaty all the time?**

○ **How does a pain reliever know which pain in your body to relieve?**

○ **Why is one of my boobs bigger than the other?**

○ **How much caffeine is too much caffeine?**

○ **Why can't I poop whenever I'm on vacation?**

And in case you're wondering, yes, we did end up writing articles that answer all of these questions, because the people need to know!

Even health editors—maybe especially health editors—have these questions. At *SELF*, we were constantly dropping weird body questions into Slack. These were people working at a wellness brand. But even we were not exempt from wondering why we're so damn gassy sometimes.

Need more proof that you're not alone? Here are some more stats you might find interesting:

○ **Most people don't even know where their heart is.** In a 2009 survey out of the UK, only 46.5 percent of people could accurately point to the location of the heart on an anatomical diagram.[4] Even fewer people could accurately point to the kidneys (42.5 percent) and the thyroid (41.8 percent). The participants in this study included 589 people from various outpatient departments in a hospital group, plus 133 people in a South London public library—so, you know, just regular people you would hope could find their heart.

○ **They also don't know where the vagina is.** A 2019 survey from YouGov found that most people really don't know their way around a vagina.[5] Of the 1,894 people who answered this question, only 48 percent could accurately label the vagina on a diagram, while only 42 percent could accurately label the urethra.

- **Most people consult Google before they consult a real doctor.** A 2019 survey conducted by the website HealthPocket polled 1,000 people in the United States between the ages of 20 and 35 and found that 79 percent of them said they would check their health problems on the internet before heading to a doctor.[6] (Honestly, same.)

It's no wonder we so often turn to Dr. Google: our general misunderstanding, shame, and embarrassment around our bodies causes us to panic about pretty much any rogue symptom.

And, you know what? I blame health class.

Health class failed us.

If you were fortunate enough to have a health class, I'm willing to bet it didn't exactly knock your socks off with useful advice for how to be a human with a body. My own health education—biology class included—was pretty useless in terms of real-world applications. I still remember that the mitochondria are the powerhouse of cells, and yet I've used that information approximately zero times since high school. Would it have been so ridiculous to spend a little less time on chlorophyll and a little more time on the digestive system? The menstrual cycle? Neurotransmitters? Literally anything that we wonder about more frequently than prokaryotes and eukaryotes?

Here's what I remember from my public school health classes—which, for reference, took place in the suburbs in Georgia between 2004 and 2007 (your mileage may vary, obviously): Learning how to put a tampon in. Watching the birth scene from the 1983 documentary *The Miracle of Life*. Looking at photos of vulvas and penises with the worst-case scenario symptoms of untreated STDs. I remember the girls getting separated from the boys for a few weeks, because God forbid we understand the ins and outs of another person's genitals, right? I remember carrying around a literal egg for a week and trying not to break it, which was my school's version of family planning. (For the record, I think I had already had sex at that point, and it is, frankly, shocking that I remembered to use a condom even though I hadn't yet experienced the trials and tribulations of egg parenthood.)

Here's what I don't remember: I don't remember ever learning what actually happens in your body during your period, or pregnancy, or arousal, or even digestion. I don't remember learning that a four-day period can be "normal" or that debilitatingly painful cramps probably aren't. I don't remember learning how things like stress, sleep, diet, and countless other factors can affect your mood and energy levels. I don't remember learning about how extremely common medications like birth control or pain relievers or antidepressants work. And I definitely don't remember learning what to do when you think something is wrong with your body.

That's why I'm not shocked that the articles I wrote got so much traffic. We're starved for basic health information.

Take a minute to think back on what you learned in health class—if you even had a health class, that is. Chances are it's wildly different from what I learned in mine. If you're having a hard time even recollecting, here are a few stories that might jog your memory:

> *"My only health class was in fifth grade, public school. We were split up by boys and girls, learned about the reproductive system and personal hygiene, and they gave us travel-size deodorants."*
>
> **—LALA J.**

> *"We had abstinence-only sex education. And they made us sign documents that said we wouldn't have sex until marriage. Except, I refused to sign mine, so they made me talk to a guidance counselor!"*
>
> **—AMY E.**

"I grew up in Togo, West Africa, and it was educational. I learned how to identify body parts, organs, systems, and certain diseases—mainly tropical diseases."

—RAYA B.

"What I remember most was handling that baby they gave us—the doll baby. We had to babysit it for a week to see what it was like to be a young parent. It cried and needed to be fed. I remember being super annoyed at having to do this task because it messed up my schedule and I had no desire to feed a crying doll in order to learn a lesson I felt I already knew—that parenting requires attention."

—ANNIE D.

"My earliest memory is from second grade but it lasted from then through the end of high school. My first memory was puppets teaching us about AIDS. They also taught us about drugs. We have a surprisingly comprehensive health class in my school district and I've found I was taught much more than my peers, including not to use two condoms at a time. They kept classes co-ed except for certain lessons. Most health classes were taught by school nurses, but one high school class was taught by a gym teacher. He had us play games like 'bowling for STDs' which were fun but actually really informative."

—KATE H.

FYI: There is no universal health education curriculum in the U.S.

Shocking, right? What we actually have are the National Health Education Standards, which were first published in 1995 and have been updated fairly regularly since then. But these standards are just what they sound like:

guidelines. Some schools meet them and some don't. Unfortunately, as of 2016, only 63 percent of public school districts had policies in place around meeting the National Health Education Standards.[7]

Another way of looking at how we're doing is to assess the percentage of schools across each state that are meeting the specific criteria laid out in those standards. To do that, I looked at the School Health Profiles 2018 report from the CDC.[8] This report includes voluntary data supplied by public schools in 43 states, 21 large urban school districts, and two territories during the 2018 spring semester. Across states, the median percentage of schools that required just one health education course in order to graduate was 40.8 percent.

Let's think about how ridiculous that is for a second. What's more crucial to both our day-to-day existence and our longevity than knowing what's going on in our bodies and how to take care of them? It's something we think about every single day—whether we're deciding what to eat or when to sleep or how to move.

Now, I understand the complexities and challenges of rolling out one universal health education curriculum to the whole country. I get that it might seem a little forced and excessive to mandate that all students in the country be taught the exact same thing. That said, what's more universal than living in a body? We all had to learn algebra—and I can guarantee you we're not all using that information equally these days.

Bottom line: Most of us didn't learn anything useful about bodies—or health, for that matter—in health class, which is a real shame since 96.9 percent of kids and teens in the United States between the ages of 7 and 17 were enrolled in school as of 2018.[9] What better opportunity exists to reach a whole group of people super eager to learn about their bodies? You truly couldn't find a more excited and engaged audience if you tried. There's really not much that's more interesting to a kid or teenager than their own changing body. Well, okay, maybe sex.

Let's (not) talk about sex.

During those BuzzFeed body brainstorms, one central theme that kept coming up was sex. Weird things our bodies do—or don't do—during sex, things we think about during sex, things that happen to our bodies before and after sex—people had a lot of sex questions. Go figure.

And that was great, because it turned out the internet had those same questions. Health articles in general made up a huge amount of BuzzFeed's traffic, but the sexual health content was the biggest slice of that, racking up millions of views per post, sometimes right after they published.

This shocked my coworkers at the time. See, BuzzFeed's whole model was built on content that gets shared widely. The point was to get content to go viral because people would share it on their pages or tag people in the comments. The website even had a formula to show writers how "shareable" their article was, based on the amount of traffic it was getting relative to how many people shared it. At the time, a few people warned me that no one was going to share an article about why you're having a hard time orgasming. And they were right—hardly anyone did! But hundreds of thousands of people clicked on the article when it was posted to one of BuzzFeed's social media pages. And that told me that people wanted more like this—even if they weren't necessarily searching for it and were way too shy to share it.

So I kept writing about boners and libido and sex dreams. And it kept going viral. This is the part of my career that my parents and journalism teachers probably aren't the proudest of. It's the part that some writers may want to bury, instead highlighting their more "serious journalism." But, to be honest, it's the time in my career when I felt most useful, most purpose-driven. I was writing about topics that people really wanted to learn more about and weren't learning about anywhere else. And I was doing it with the same rigor I used when reporting on any other health topic—digging through peer-reviewed research, translating barely readable recommendations from major medical organizations, and interviewing renowned experts in the fields of gynecology, urology, and psychology.

I'll never forget one comment I read on one of my articles: *This article taught me more than sex ed ever did.*

And that's exactly why I was doing it. If you think a lack of universal health education is bonkers, forget about universal sex education.

Let's look back at the sex education data from the School Health Profiles 2018 report. The median percentage of high schools that taught the benefits of being sexually abstinent was 93 percent, while only 62.1 percent taught how to correctly use a condom. Looking at middle schools, the median percentage of schools that taught students how to correctly use a condom was just 27.6 percent. And the median percentage of schools in which the lead health education teacher had received professional development in the last two years about teaching students of different sexual orientations and gender identities was just 32.5 percent.[10]

It was obvious why people were clicking on my articles. They weren't getting comprehensive, inclusive sex education anywhere else.

One of the experts I called on a lot during that time was Logan Levkoff, PhD, a renowned sex educator and author based in New York City. As a sex educator, she spends a lot of her time speaking with young adults in school about sex. And whenever we talk, I'm reminded of just how subpar my own sex education was.

"I like having all genders—regardless of someone's assigned sex—to be in a classroom together. And the reason for that is that regardless of whether we're assigned male, female, intersex, our bodies are pretty much the same, they are just arranged in different ways. But this idea that you have to have a certain body part to hear about something seems just ridiculous to me, mostly because the changes that we experience, for the most part, are really similar. And if things are different, then they're all happening for the same reasons, which is to activate your reproductive system, or to give your body certain choices and options for the future," explains Levkoff.

Think about all the times that someone of a different gender was shocked or confused by something totally unremarkable going on with your own body. Think about how much better our understanding of our bodies would be if we all learned about all of our parts. Together, even! I know. So scandalous.

Levkoff gave me a perfect example of this that happened in one of her classes. She was speaking to a seventh grade class of mixed genders when a boy in the class asked, "What happens if you're having sex and someone gets their period?" A valid question for a seventh grader, to be honest, and a great thing to discuss openly with all genders—rather than tailoring your message in any particular way.

"The assumption was there was something wrong with it," says Levkoff. "And I said, 'Well, guess what, some bodies menstruate. So might that happen? Sure. Might there be some couples who are completely okay with that? Sure. Might there be some couples who are uncomfortable with that? Sure.'"

The point she was trying to make was this: Bodily functions like that are part and parcel of having a body. You're allowed to feel however you want to feel about period sex, but if someone's body randomly decides to menstruate while you're having sex, that's not bad or abnormal or harmful. It just means you'll probably have to do laundry sooner than you'd planned.

I wish more of us had been told— often—that our bodies were normal, our questions were normal, our curiosities were normal.

"Certain bodies ejaculate semen. Certain bodies menstruate. These things just happen. And that's okay. They're supposed to happen," says Levkoff.

Listen, I know that might sound totally simplistic to some of you, but for so many of us, information about our bodies was not doled out in that simple, straightforward, no-big-deal way. And I really wish it had been. I wish more

> *We don't have to have all the answers. But we do need to have the space and the courage to ask questions. I promise, you aren't the only one with your question.*

of us had been told—often—that our bodies were normal, our questions were normal, our curiosities were normal. Imagine how much more confident and less confused we would all be.

"I think that young people—if you give them the skills to do these things and the information—have absolutely no problem doing it, which is incredible," says Levkoff. "I think that when we are askable and open adults that are nonjudgmental and acknowledge that it's okay to have a lot of questions about a lot of things, then we become the type of people who they'll ask questions to freely. And they won't feel shame in asking them, because they know that part of being a human being is having lots of questions."

Heads-up that this is going to be a theme in the book: the power and importance of asking questions. Whether you're 17 or 70, this is a lesson I want to you to remember: We don't have to have all the answers. But we do need to have the space and the courage to ask questions. I promise, you aren't the only one with your question.

We have a health literacy problem.

We've established that most of us didn't learn squat about our bodies in school, but that's not the only reason that it's so hard for us to navigate health questions out in the real world. It's one thing when we can't tell our vagina from our vulva, but when it comes to understanding basic health information, that's just the tip of the iceberg. We have a health literacy problem, folks.

If you've never heard of health literacy, that's okay. I'm sure you're actually familiar with the concept even if you don't know it yet. *Health literacy* is defined as "the degree to which individuals have the capacity to obtain, process, and understand basic health information and services needed to make appropriate health decisions." I know that's a lot to take in, but stay with me. That's the definition of health literacy developed for the Current Bibliographies in Medicine back in 2000, but this concept has been defined in many different ways by many different groups over the years.[11]

I'm not going to attempt to cover all of the various definitions and explanations of health literacy here. Instead, I'll tell you what *I* mean when I say health literacy. To me, health literacy is having a good-enough understanding of our bodies and our health and a good idea of where to go for answers if we still have questions. Health literacy is what's needed to navigate the health care system a little more easily and to process all the health messages we're getting from friends, doctors, the news, social media, etc. Health literacy means that you have the basic knowledge, tools, and know-how to make informed decisions about your health. That's what I mean when I talk about health literacy.

Let's go over some examples in your everyday life where health literacy comes into play:

- When you're reading the label on a new prescription

- When you're trying to pick a cold medicine from a shelf with 73 different kinds

- When you see an anti-smoking commercial on TV or calorie counts on a menu (rude, by the way)

- When you get the test results of your Pap smear, mammogram, colonoscopy, etc.

- When you try to remember when you're actually supposed to get a Pap smear, mammogram, colonoscopy, etc.

- When you're talking to a nurse about what hurts

- When your doctor says your blood pressure is a little high

- When you make literally any choice that relates to your body or your health

Health literacy is your ability to navigate these everyday situations—or not. I see it as the skills needed to narrow that gap between what the average person with a body knows and what health care professionals know.

There's another explanation of health literacy in the Current Bibliographies of Medicine in 2000 that I find especially profound, particularly for anyone living with a chronic illness: "Health literacy problems have grown as patients are asked to assume more responsibility for self-care in a complex health care system. Patients' health literacy, then, can be thought of as the currency needed to negotiate this complex system." Unfortunately, way too many people don't have this necessary currency—and that's a systemic problem, not a personal failing.

By one estimate, nearly 9 out of 10 adults have difficulty using everyday health information—like the kind of messages you get in a doctor's office, in a drugstore, or in the media.[12] As I write this book, currently surrounded by confusing, conflicting, and constantly updating information about COVID-19, I'm left wondering who that 1 person out of 10 is who *doesn't* find this difficult. Because this is really fucking difficult.

But, once again, it's not your fault.

There are a lot of factors that stand in the way of health literacy. And once I explain them, you're probably going to be shaking your fist like, "Ugh, yes, that *is* annoying! Why *don't* they fix that!?" Because these are things you encounter *every single day,* but you probably don't think about how they're affecting the way you think about your body or the decisions you make about your health.

We already covered a big one: the lack of consistent, comprehensive health education to give us even a baseline understanding of our bodies, not to mention any key health markers we should know about. I think we can all agree that better health education across the board would go a long way when it comes to making decisions about our health.

But there's more than that.

Most of the need-to-know health information that comes from legit, reputable sources is really difficult to understand. And when something is too hard to understand, we tend to just ignore it and get our information somewhere else.

"Health literacy problems have grown as patients are asked to assume more responsibility for self-care in a complex health care system. Patients' health literacy, then, can be thought of as the currency needed to negotiate this complex system."

Unnecessary medical jargon is a real problem when it comes to health literacy. And you can find this jargon pretty much everywhere—on a medical website, on your prescription bottle, in paperwork you get from your doctor's office, or even in a conversation with your health care provider. I'm pretty used to it after reporting on health and health care issues for so many years, but my eyes still glaze over sometimes when I'm reading something that just doesn't feel accessible to people who aren't medical professionals.

To find out more about this, I talked to Rima Rudd, ScD, a renowned leader in health literacy studies and senior lecturer on health literacy, education, and policy at Harvard's T.H. Chan School of Public Health.

"Medicine, nursing, public health, epidemiology, all science—we all use a certain amount of jargon that we've been trained for in school. And so we're talking amongst ourselves and we're not necessarily talking to the public," explains Rudd. "So our writing is not good for public consumption. It's not clear. It's filled with jargon. It's filled with words that are not defined. It's filled with charts and graphs that are not clear to the average citizen."

That's one of the reasons why it's so hard to measure health literacy— it's not enough to say, "Well, people obviously just don't know enough about health, so that's why they don't understand this." Actually, maybe we're just making health messaging harder than it needs to be.

"If you give someone a text that's extraordinarily difficult and filled with jargon, they're going to have difficulty with that text. So you can fix it in two ways: You can improve the literacy skills of the public, which could take a very long time," says Rudd. "And you can improve the materials. Make it easier to understand, clarify, offer explanations."

For instance, here are a few examples of some medical jargon that is majorly unhelpful to the average person, along with a more conversational way of explaining it:

IDIOPATHIC = when something has an unknown cause

COMORBIDITY = when someone has two different conditions at the same time (like anxiety and depression)

CONTRAINDICATION = when a certain treatment isn't recommended because it could be harmful

PROGNOSIS = the likely outcome of someone's disease

SUBLINGUAL = a medication you take under your tongue

See, it's not hard to imagine a situation where your doctor rattles off a few of these words or you read them online and you're left wondering what the hell you're supposed to do with that information. Again, it's not the patient's fault, and it's often not even the doctor's fault. But we need to recognize that this exchange of information—and pretty crucial information in this case—hinges on both people understanding what we're talking about.

"Literacy is an interaction," says Rudd. "It's an interaction between a person and a text, between a speaker and a listener, between the designer and the person who's using a particular product. It's always an interaction."

As a health editor, a lot of my job was about easing that interaction by translating this medical jargon into something more conversational yet still accurate. It's tricky and it's time-consuming, but I did it because I want as many people as possible to have access to important, accurate material about their health. I love calling up experts and talking to them about a complicated issue, then distilling that information into text that people will actually understand—maybe even enjoy and share. That's one small aspect of health literacy that I feel like I can help with.

But I can't be there in the doctor's office with you when you're scared and vulnerable, feet in the stirrups, covered up by, essentially, a paper towel. I can't be there when your doctor asks if you have any questions, and you know you do but you're not really sure what they are or how to ask them. I can't be there when you're on the phone with your insurance company for hours and it still feels like you're speaking two different languages—or maybe you actually are.

See, health information that is clear and helpful is just one part of the puzzle. There are so many other pieces.

Cynthia Baur, PhD, has spent her career examining all of the pieces that go into this puzzle. As the senior advisor for health literacy at the CDC, she created the CDC's health literacy website and cocreated the CDC's Clear Communication Index, a tool to help craft public health information that people can actually understand. Now, she's the director of the Horowitz Center for Health Literacy at University of Maryland.

When we spoke, Baur explained to me that while clear health messages are obviously important, there are so many other factors that dictate whether or not we're going to actually absorb and act on the information we receive.

Attention is one factor. We can teach doctors and health organizations to put out messages that are written for regular people, but how do we get people to pay attention to them?

Relevancy is another. I can have access to messages about what a Pap smear is and why I need one, but if I'm currently without a job or without health insurance, getting a Pap smear might be far down on my list of priorities.

The complexity of our health care system is also a huge consideration. We can have clear, actionable, relevant information right in our faces, but if there are all sorts of obstacles in the way of acting on it, that's a problem.

"We've built this thing called the health care system. Nobody really knows how it all works at the end of the day," says Baur. "You encounter this very complicated thing only a couple of times a year or under great duress— like when you're not feeling well, you're emotionally compromised, you're in pain, and all those other things. It's just no surprise that it doesn't go as well as people would expect."

Addressing health literacy isn't simply about changing the message—it's also about dismantling the obstacles that stand in the way of someone acting on that message.

"I think clear messages are important," she says. "I teach a lot of people how to do that. At the same time, I feel like if we don't change fundamentally how health care services are organized and delivered, all of my clear messages will still only get us so far. They will not create a health literate society."

And, finally, we have to remember that the conversations happening around health and health literacy aren't happening in a vacuum. What's going on in the world—in politics, media, social justice movements, public health— all impact how people receive and respond to health information.

"These are very precarious times," says Rudd. "When people are talking about alternative facts, when people are talking about beliefs rather than findings, when scientists' voices are muddled or excluded from the room, we're in trouble."

Like I said, we have a health literacy problem, and it's caused by a tangled web of frustrating factors that many of us are way too familiar with at this point. It's the comprehensive health education that we're not getting. It's the policies and politics that dictate what we're taught, what we're told, and what choices we have in our health care. It's the jargon-filled materials that we have no clue what to do with and the frustrating interactions with medical staff that leave us feeling confused and discouraged. It's the incredibly complex health care system that makes it so damn hard to access basic care. It's the fact that all of this takes a lot of work, and most people don't have the time or the resources or the patience to figure it out.

It's no wonder that we go searching for answers to our questions that are simpler, easier, more immediate. The problem is, there is so, so much information out there—each article, video, and social media post contradicting the next—and most people don't know who or what to trust.

We also have a media literacy problem.

While I'm over here making up my ideal high school curriculum, I'm going to suggest one more class that I see as a necessity for any person with a body and access to the media in some shape or form. We need to teach people media literacy.

As with health literacy, it's hard to pin down a concise definition of what media literacy encompasses. But the National Association for Media Literacy Education does a pretty good job: "Media literacy is the ability to access, analyze, evaluate, create, and act using all forms of communication."[13]

Again, media literacy is multifaceted and I'm not going to cover all the nuances in this chapter. But let's talk about just how necessary it is to have a good working knowledge of your body and your health.

Think about it: Where do you get the bulk of your health information? With the exception of people in the medical profession, I'm guessing most people get most of their health content from the media. Maybe you get nutrition and workout advice from a magazine, you read about a new health study on Facebook, you stay updated on the pandemic from the news, and when you have a random health question, you consult the internet.

That's why media literacy is so important when it comes to your health: We're constantly bombarded by tons of information from all different types of media. But the unfortunate reality is that not all media is accurate.

And I'm not just talking about fake health news (which, ugh, is really a thing). I'm also talking about health news that's sloppy, biased, not well reported, not well sourced, or not telling the whole story. And don't even get me started on the health media that's just trying to sell you something.

"You really need to develop a healthy dose of skepticism about things that you come across either through internet search or that somebody shares with you on a social media site," says Baur. "People should just be far less accepting of that content. And until people start developing that more critical lens for what they find online, I don't know how we're going to really get people to not just take the things that turn up on the first page of the results."

So what does it look like to have a healthy dose of skepticism? Here are a few basic ground rules, which I'll go over in more depth in chapter 5.

○ **Know how to spot a legitimate source of health information. A few well-known ones are:**
  - The CDC
  - The World Health Organization
  - The National Institutes of Health
  - A medical professional who specializes in the topic being discussed and has the necessary credentials to prove it.

○ **If you come across interesting health information anywhere else, check the sources. They should be using some combination of the legitimate sources above.**

○ **If something sounds too good to be true, it probably is. I know, it sucks, I'm sorry. But it's true. In this case, checking the information against multiple sources is a pretty good way to go.**

○ **If anyone ever says "research shows . . .," you better be able to see that research. Bonus points if they sum it up for you, but they should point you in the direction of the actual research paper, too.**

I know, this sounds exhausting, but as with anything, the more you flex this muscle, the stronger and more second nature it'll become.

Okay, so that was a lot.

I don't say all of this to scare you. Instead, I say it to empower you. If you, like me, tend to catastrophize any little thing that's happening in your body, it's not your fault. We're working with a pretty sad amount of information about the way our bodies work.

And when we don't know how something is supposed to look, feel, or smell, we often end up turning to the quickest and easiest resource at our disposal: the internet.

Enter Google.

So, the internet says you're either pregnant or dying.

I'LL NEVER FORGET READING SOMETHING SOMEWHERE ON the internet that convinced me I was pregnant. Actually, let me be more specific, because that happened a lot.

In this particular instance I was 19 and wondering where the hell my period was. It seemed like I had gotten it the day before, but then it just . . . disappeared.

Well that seems bad, I thought.

While I've never particularly loved bleeding from my vagina, there's a certain comfort in that monthly annoyance when you're a 19-year-old who is irrationally afraid of getting pregnant. So you can imagine my surprise when, instead of my regularly scheduled five days of bleeding, all I got was one tiny tampon's worth of blood followed by several days of panic.

I was on a birth control pill, so pregnancy was unlikely, but that meant nothing to me at that moment. To be honest, I can't even remember now if I had had sex that month. Again, irrelevant. My period was ghosting me, and therefore I was almost definitely pregnant.

As one does when one's period is wonky, I consulted Google, which told me there are all sorts of reasons why I might have a very light, almost non-existent period. My eyes scanned the page, searching for confirmation of my anxiety and finally settling on the closest thing: some people experience implantation bleeding when a fertilized egg attaches to the uterine lining, so a small amount of blood could actually be a sign of pregnancy.

WELP, THERE IT IS. DEFINITELY PREGNANT. NO OTHER POSSIBLE CONCLUSION.

Eventually, I went to see my gynecologist and explained the whole ordeal: My period came and went in a matter of hours. Why was it so weird and light? What did I do wrong? I was definitely pregnant, right?

She looked back at my chart and reminded me that I had been on the same birth control pill for four years. One possibility was that my period just gradually became lighter and easier to deal with as a result of the birth control—a common side effect. Another possibility was that any number of factors could have thrown off my period that month—like stress, lack of sleep, and the complete chaos of starting college. Sure, pregnancy *could* be a possibility, but it was a very unlikely one in my case—made even more unlikely by the negative pregnancy test I took.

So I had an answer—a more thorough and less terrifying one than the internet gave me. And you'd think I would have learned my lesson about turning to Dr. Google in times of distress. But of course I didn't.

Why are we like this?

Why we can't stop Googling our symptoms—even when we know better

When I first sat down and asked myself—and the experts—why we put ourselves through the search engine ringer even when it almost never ends well, I expected the answer to be as simple as: because we can.

After all, we are nothing if not instant gratification–seekers. While 10 years ago we might have sat around with our friends arguing for half an hour about the band that sang that song in that commercial, now we can simply whip out our phones and see who is right within seconds. Nothing makes me feel older than lamenting how kids today will never know what it's like to not be able to type something into a search engine and get an instant answer. (Whether that answer will be right, of course, is an issue for another chapter.)

So I expected our constant symptom-Googling to be just another by-product of the limitless information at our fingertips. But, of course, it's more complicated than that. Here's the moment when Abramowitz broke it down for me: "There is some short-term escape that people anticipate getting: 'I'm going to look this up and then I'm going to know for sure! I'm going to figure it out!' We know from research that folks with health anxiety often have an intolerance of uncertainty. You don't like not knowing."

At this point I actually had to stifle a laugh, because yes, this is me—with uncertainty about my health or my job or my relationships, I find it all completely unbearable and will do just about anything to try to gain some certainty. And yes, often that involves consulting the internet to see if I can get some answers.

"The person has some sort of expectation that it's going to make them feel better. In the short term sometimes it does; in the long run it just makes things worse. But we, as humans, we go for the short-term anxiety reduction."

So it's not just the availability of this information that makes it so irresistible. It's our fear and anxiety that cause us to seek reassurance wherever and however we can get it.

"Even if it's short-lived, it's something. It's better than living with uncertainty," says Abramowitz. (Oh, you mean living with, "It's *probably* nothing?")

As a result, many of us have actually conditioned ourselves to whip out our phones when we're feeling concerned about our bodies. When we're plagued with that confusion and uncertainty, we want to make those feelings go away. So we look around at the tools we have at our disposal, and often the closest and simplest one is the internet. Sometimes we find information that's genuinely helpful and empathetic, which makes us less anxious, less scared, and more able to move on with our lives. Looking our problem up helped, which means we're pretty likely to do it again when we find ourselves in a similar bind. Of course, other times our search results just leave us even more stressed than we were in the first place. But, somehow, that doesn't stop us from trying again and hoping for a different outcome.

This is a great example of operant conditioning, a principle of psychology that explains how our behavior can be influenced by stimulus-response patterns that either reinforce or discourage a particular behavior. To put it a little more simply: Googling our symptoms is a lot like gambling. Let me explain.

I first learned about operant conditioning, a term coined by psychologist B.F. Skinner, in a college course I took called Conditioning and Learning.[14] I needed a lab class to graduate with my psych degree, and it sounded interesting enough. What I didn't realize until the first day was that we would be dealing with *literal lab rats* to learn these principles. The whole thing was a PETA nightmare, but the lessons stuck with me.

Operant conditioning says that our behavior is conditioned by reinforcements (a good consequence that makes us more likely to repeat the behavior) or punishments (a bad consequence that makes us less likely to repeat the behavior). Both reinforcements and punishments can be either positive or negative—in this case, meaning that something is added (positive) or taken away (negative).

Here's an example to show the difference between positive and negative reinforcement, both of which would make you *more* likely to repeat the behavior:

- Positive reinforcement: You walked the dog, and you got $20. (The *addition* of a good stimulus reinforces the behavior.)

- Negative reinforcement: The dog stopped begging when you took him for a walk. (The *removal* of an annoying stimulus reinforces the behavior.)

How does this explain why we keep going back to Google when we're stressing about our bodies? "We would call it negative reinforcement. Which means that the behavior of looking stuff up is increased because you're removing an aversive stimulus, which is the feelings of anxiety," says Abramowitz.

But since we don't always get that removal of anxiety, another facet of operant conditioning comes into play: the reinforcement schedule. Skinner theorized that it's not just how but also *when* you get reinforcement that impacts how likely you are to keep doing something. Consider a slot machine. Sometimes when you put money in and pull the lever, you're rewarded with more money—thus the behavior is positively reinforced. But other times you put money in, pull the lever, and you lose it all—thus the behavior is punished. So why do we keep gambling? It's the same reason we keep looking up our symptoms online even though it rarely makes us feel better: because *sometimes* we win.

If you played the slot machine and won every single time, chances are you'd keep playing. If you played and lost every single time, chances are you'd stop playing. But what if you sometimes won and sometimes lost, and you had no idea when either was going to happen? That's what Skinner would call variable ratio reinforcement: when you get a desired outcome after an unpredictable amount of tries. That unpredictability is what makes this behavior so hard to quit. You keep coming back for more, because you hope that this time you'll get the desired outcome.

So, in a sense, Googling our symptoms is a lot like gambling. Sometimes we're rewarded, and we close the laptop feeling confident and calmer. Other times we visit site after site, our anxiety building with every possibility we read about. But as long as our uncertainty is occasionally eased by this behavior, we'll keep going back to it and hope for the best.

As Abramowitz explained, this anticipated short-term gain is incredibly tempting. We think we'll get some answers without having to do a whole lot—like take off work, leave our house, talk to a real human, pay out of pocket, or—if we're fortunate—shell out a copay, run some tests, and maybe the most dreaded of all, *wait*.

There is nothing easy about accessing medical care. And that's not to mention that your ability to access and afford that care varies widely depending on your circumstances. Even in the best-case scenario—you're insured and you have the understanding and resources to know where to go to get this question answered—you still need to:

1. Find a doctor or specialist that you can get to.

2. Make sure they're in-network for your insurance.

3. Wait who-knows-how-long for an appointment.

4. Make sure you can actually be available to attend that appointment.

5 Articulate your concerns to the nurse or doctor in a brief but thorough manner (since they have roughly four minutes to see you).

6 Hope that the doctor takes your concerns seriously and has some information for you.

7 Pay for your visit—regardless of whether or not your issue was resolved.

8 Pray that whatever prescriptions they ordered aren't too expensive.

9 Take their advice and hope for the best.

And at the end of all of that, if the first course of treatment didn't really help, you're right back where you started.

It's no wonder that we're tempted by the instant answers we *could* have if we're just brave enough to type what we're feeling into that search bar. But what happens next?

HOW GETTING HEALTH CARE IS LIKE GOING TO THE GROCERY STORE IN A PANDEMIC

Navigating the health care system can be scary, frustrating, and confusing even for those of us who are the most prepared, most informed, and most fortunate. It can be downright terrifying for everyone else.

Cynthia Baur, PhD, shared with me an example that she recently posed to a room full of researchers and clinicians: "Imagine if we ran grocery stores like we ran health care. Imagine that you drove up and you got out and you walked in and you didn't know what was going to be available. You didn't know how much it was going to cost. You didn't know how long it would take you to go through the store. You didn't know what you would walk out with when you were done. How excited would you be to go to the grocery store? You wouldn't want to go."

Several weeks after I spoke with Baur, I was reminded of that example when I went to the grocery store in New York City for the first time since COVID-19 had been declared a pandemic. Baur's words suddenly felt more like a prophecy than a metaphor, because shopping for essentials was now a scary, confusing, frustrating experience—one in which you were going in blind, not sure what you were going to get, how long it was going to take, or how much it was going to cost. It felt a bit like trying to navigate health care under normal circumstances.

But I had options. I could pay a premium for a grocery delivery service. I could go during off-peak hours because I had a flexible job that allowed me to work safely from home. I could have friends ship me disinfecting wipes. And I was reminded that, when things are awful, things aren't the same level of awful for everyone.

The reality is that there is an endless stream of barriers to accessing health care in the United States, and those barriers disproportionately harm women, LGBTQ+ folks, Black and Indigenous people and other people of color, and immigrants. And the more barriers you encounter on that journey, the harder it will be to access necessary—even life-saving—care. Those barriers include the obvious, like having health insurance, but they also cover the countless other obstacles that most people never think about if they aren't things that affect them, like:

- Living far from the nearest medical center—let alone the nearest specialist

- Not being able to take off work, coordinate childcare, and/or find reliable transportation to your appointments

- Having a language barrier that makes every single step of the process that much more difficult

- Knowing that you likely won't be able to afford the medical bills when they come, even though you have no idea how much they'll be

- Growing up in a family, community, or culture that distrusts mainstream American medical care

- A previous experience with trauma, stigma, shame, embarrassment, misdiagnoses, or even issues of consent in a medical setting

Okay, so you did it. You Googled your symptoms. Now what?

Listen, I don't expect—nor do I want—you to never look up your health questions again. We both know you're going to continue searching your symptoms, and to be completely honest, I know I will, too. As I explained above, it's totally reasonable to want to get quick answers for a body concern, question, or curiosity. I get it.

But, as I'm sure you know, it's also really common to come out of that search feeling way more panicked than you did when you went in. You're now convinced that your anxious thoughts or fears were totally warranted. Maybe you even picked up a few more along the way.

As someone who knows a lot about the way health content is created and distributed online, I also know exactly why this happens. Better yet, I'm confident that once *you* know more about the way this stuff gets made, you'll get a lot better at distinguishing between what's helpful and what's all hype, too.

So I'm going to outline some of the most common symptom-searching scenarios that often feed into health anxiety and body stress. If you're someone who tends to Google your symptoms or health questions, the following are going to look really familiar to you. But what's new is the *context* that will help you become a lot calmer and more conscientious in these scenarios in the future.

THE SIGNS AND SYMPTOMS ARTICLE

We've all had it at some point. And no, I'm not talking about HPV (although, yes, we've all probably had that at some point, too). We've all gotten what I call the "yep, dying" search result. It's the one where you Google your symptoms and get an answer that seems completely out of proportion to what you expected. But also, *could it be that?!*

This answer is usually in the form of a listicle that tells you your innocuous symptom can be caused by such a laughably long list of factors that it's neither helpful nor reassuring. Sure, that stomach pain could be indigestion. Or it could be norovirus, IBS, Crohn's disease, kidney stones, your appendix bursting, or 12 other very scary-sounding possibilities.

This is one of the most stressful things about consulting the internet for a health problem: the fact that *all* of the options are laid out with almost equal weight and no regard for your unique situation.

I call these signs and symptoms articles, and they're pretty much the bread and butter of digital health content. They get a ton of traffic from searches, because people are always looking up things like "signs of a heart attack" or "stomach pain." I've written and edited a lot of these articles, and I do think they can be genuinely helpful and informative. But they can also be pretty major offenders of fearmongering if they aren't written responsibly.

You've definitely seen—and probably clicked on—a few signs and symptoms articles. Things like:

○ **13 Sneaky Signs of Breast Cancer**

○ **15 Common Causes of Night Sweats**

○ **23 Stomach Symptoms You Shouldn't Ignore**

I'm sure you can see how, if you're already feeling anxious about one of these things, reading an article with a title like this could send you spiraling. (Editing them sure did, too!)

The reason these articles are so long and exhaustive isn't because it's all relevant to your situation—it's because that helps them rank higher in Google's search results. Whether an article is on the first page or the seventh page of the search results likely depends on a few different factors, like when it was published, how thorough it is, how closely the site's content matches what you searched for, and even how authoritative and trustworthy Google considers that article.[15] Essentially, content creators are incentivized to write health articles that are good quality, yes, but also strategically formatted in a way that Google will find worthy. They know that the more causes of stomach pain they add to the list, the higher up it could be in the search results, which translates to more people clicking and more eyes on the page. And, without getting too deep in the weeds here, most websites are always aiming for more visitors to their pages and more time spent on those pages, because that translates to advertising dollars.

When you land on one of these articles, it's really easy to zero in on the worst-case scenario and assume that's what you're dealing with, especially if you're someone who is prone to health anxiety.

Abramowitz blames this on confirmation bias: "When we start to believe something, when we start to be afraid of something, we look for evidence to confirm our fears." He gives the example of typing "stomach pain" into the search bar and landing on a long list of possible culprits—many of which are benign or no big deal. And yet we choose to focus on the scariest, most serious one.

I am notorious for this. I even do this when I'm *editing* a signs and symptoms article! I once edited an article about reasons why you're waking up a lot in the middle of the night and convinced myself that I had sleep apnea, a thyroid condition, and type 2 diabetes. Not one of them—all of them!

If you also tend to latch on to the most stressful possibility when reading a health article, it doesn't mean you have to avoid these articles entirely. It just means that you should be aware of the limitations that come with consulting the internet about your symptoms. Yes, you'll probably get some answers to your questions, but you won't get every answer to every question. And the answers won't be unique to you. In fact, they'll be specifically designed to apply to a broad range of people. When you ask the internet what's up with this random boob pain, you're going to get a laundry list of possible culprits ranging from no big deal to very big deal—and at least nine others in between. You probably know nothing about the writer of this article, just as they know nothing about you or your boobs. Remember that the next time you read a signs and symptoms article and assume the worst.

THE TERRIFYING CASE REPORT YOU'LL NEVER FORGET

Woman finds worms in her eye.[16] Man dies after eating old pasta.[17] Okay, I'm going to stop now because I'm starting to freak myself out.

These are examples of headlines covering medical case reports. A case report is a detailed paper where experts share in-depth information about a particular patient, sometimes in a scientific journal. It's essentially a scientific study of one specific phenomenon occurring in one particular individual or setting. Because it's so specific, it obviously doesn't give you any generalizable findings, but they're useful for other reasons—like furthering a new hypothesis or inspiring new research. Basically they're helpful to researchers, but not so much to the general public.

I totally get why case reports are useful, and yet, they're one of my least favorite things on the internet. That's because they spread like wildfire. Digital journalists—eager to hit their quotas—feel compelled to report on them. Readers—drawn in by a truly WTF headline—can't help but click and share them. The problem is, a case report is a case report for a reason. It's talking about a *rare* medical phenomenon, and researchers are documenting it and analyzing it *because* it's so rare. Unfortunately, when a case report gets shared by everyone and their mom on Facebook, it starts to seem anything but rare. It starts to seem like a legit thing you need to worry about.

Let me tell you about a particularly embarrassing time this happened to me. One day at work I saw a story trending online about a college student who had died after eating old leftovers—a thing that I, and most people, do all the damn time. I avoided clicking on it, knowing that it would most likely trigger my anxiety, but I finally caved after I saw it covered by a dozen different outlets.

The story goes like this: A 20-year-old college student reheated some spaghetti with tomato sauce that he had made five days before but left in the kitchen at room temperature.[18] After eating it, he went off to play sports but came home just 30 minutes later with a headache, stomach pain, and nausea, which eventually gave way to vomiting and diarrhea. The next morning, his parents found him dead. Although the autopsy was inconclusive, an investigation pointed to an infection of *Bacillus cereus,* a bacteria that can lead to food poisoning, which in this case was thought to be the most likely cause of death. The *Business Insider* article I was reading said the infection was sometimes referred to as "fried rice syndrome," since the bacteria is known to grow on rice left out at room temperature for too long.

All of this was detailed in a case report in the *Journal of Clinical Microbiology,* because—as we can all agree—this is pretty shocking stuff that scientists would want to document and learn more about.

So back to me—reading this with a clenched jaw and wide eyes in my office, then closing the tab and trying to push it from my memory. Fastforward about two weeks later, and I'm at home on a Saturday afternoon, getting some work done. I reheated some leftovers from two nights before— spicy fried rice from a Thai restaurant nearby. It tasted a little weird, but I had never reheated leftovers from this place before, so I figured it just wasn't as fresh reheated. After a few minutes, I noticed there were a lot of onions in the dish . . . and I had specifically asked for no onions in my fried rice. That's when I realized that these were not my leftovers from two nights prior. These were someone else's leftovers . . . from at least a week prior.

FRIED RICE SYNDROME. It was the first thought that popped into my head, followed quickly by *OMG I'm gonna puke and then probably die.* I immediately spit the onion-filled mouthful back into the bowl, threw the whole thing away, and then paced back and forth in my apartment trying to figure out what to do. I searched around online to find the stories again, trying to determine my odds of dying from this very old fried rice sitting in my stomach. It didn't help. I was getting more and more nauseous by the minute but unable to pin it on the rice *or* my steadily increasing anxiety.

I called my friend, an emergency department nurse, and asked her if I should make myself throw up. She said definitely don't do that and told me I'd be fine.

Not satisfied with that answer, I asked another friend's husband who happens to be a gastroenterologist. He, too, said not to worry about it.

"But what about *Bacillus cereus*?! This case report I read . . ." He kindly cut me off by reminding me that case reports are case reports *because* they're rare—rare enough to be documented in a scientific journal. If I felt sick—or got sick—I could go to the doctor and explain what had happened. Until then, I should try to calm down and not think about it.

As you can see, case reports are like horror movies for people with health anxiety. They tell a terrifying story that haunts you long after it's over because it seems like something that could totally happen to you—even if the chances of it actually happening to you are incredibly slim or even basically impossible. According to Abramowitz, the tendency to overestimate risk is common in people with anxiety, which makes sense. We tend to focus on those worst-case scenarios. And that's exactly what happens when we read a scary case report—it sticks in our memory and we overestimate the risk that it poses to us.

I knew all of this, and still I fell victim to the case report spiral. Why? Because when you see a story over and over again, you're more likely to remember it and believe it.

"There's a phenomenon called the availability bias. This is our tendency to get fooled into thinking because we hear a lot about something that it's actually more prevalent," explains Abramowitz.

This death-by-leftovers story was all over my feeds in January 2019. I follow a lot of health brands, but still—it was everywhere. And here's the most irritating part: the actual case report was published way back in 2011! The story seemed to have resurfaced because of a YouTube video dramatizing the report, which went up in January 2019, causing tons of outlets to report on it like it was news.[19] As a journalist, I get it: Imagine being an underpaid online writer who has to meet a ridiculous production or traffic quota each week. You see a story about a guy who died after eating five-day-old pasta and you're probably thinking *jackpot*.

But as a health journalist who also suffers from health anxiety, I get frustrated when I see this. Choosing to publish a story is choosing to tell your audience that this is something they should care about. And hey, there's an argument to be made that reading about this eight-year-old case report is something people should care about—if only to be reminded of the importance of food safety practices. But when it's reported in a way that's fearmongering, as it often was in this case, with no explanation of how rare it actually is to have your organs shut down as a result of this particular type of food poisoning, it's just sloppy reporting and careless editing. Even worse, it can make some people (*raises hand*) even more anxious.

Which brings me to the next common culprit that often fuels our health anxiety . . .

THE RABBIT HOLE OF INFORMATION AND MISINFORMATION

This is probably the most likely scenario that happens when you head online with a health question—whether you're wondering about a symptom, a new diagnosis, or just a random body curiosity. You type in something pretty general—let's say "thinning hair"—and you get 2 billion search results. So helpful! Not at all excessive and overwhelming!

Maybe from there you start narrowing things down:

○ **"Causes of thinning hair"** (7.6 million results)

○ **"Treatments for thinning hair"** (19.3 million results)

○ **"Thinning hair in my 20s help"** (16.5 million results)

The sheer amount of health information available online is exciting but also exhausting. It feels like if you just keep reading, keep scrolling, keep clicking, you'll find the answer you're looking for.

But the biggest issue with health information on the internet isn't the quantity—it's the quality. I write health content, and I'll be the first one to tell you that it's not all good out there. There's no widespread quality control for all of the content published online, and the unfortunate reality is that the hype is often sexier than the truth. Someone who calls themself a health coach, with 200,000 followers and a blue checkmark on Instagram, is probably going to reach a lot more people with their content than the CDC.

Hype is often sexier than the truth . . .

The possibility of stumbling upon completely inaccurate health information online is, unfortunately, very high.

Even reputable, well-meaning media brands are occasionally guilty of clickbait headlines and surface-level reporting that can be misleading or confusing—like the unnecessarily fearmongering "7 Common Symptoms That Might Be Cancer" or "Super Gonorrhea Is Here and It's Spreading." Headlines like these aren't just annoying and irresponsible, they also contribute to the confusion and stress that we have about our bodies.

As a writer and editor, I know why these articles run and why these headlines get approved. Most media companies are under mounting pressure to cut costs while increasing production and traffic. The result: grabby headlines that only tell half the story and brief articles lacking the necessary nuance.

For all of these reasons, I like to tell people that going online for health answers is a lot like going online to buy a house. It's a great place to start because you can cast a really wide net, but you'll probably need to filter out a lot of noise that doesn't apply to you before you can begin to find the stuff that does. You'll have to watch out for misleading information and straight-up scams. And, finally, after tons of searching and open tabs, you'll either give up in frustration or you'll find that you're actually a lot more confident in your next steps. But, in all likelihood, you're not going to finish your journey online—meaning, you're probably not going to buy a house, sight unseen, on the internet. Just like you're probably not going to get a definitive diagnosis or clear-cut answer to your unique health question online.

Obviously this isn't an exhaustive list of what can happen when you go looking for health answers online. But the end result is usually the same: You're just as scared, confused, and stressed out as you were before. Armed with a whole lot of information that may or may not be helpful, where do you go next? For many of us, to whatever wellness fad or fast fix is currently trending.

CHAPTER 3

CBD oil, cleanses, jade eggs, and other things your body probably doesn't need

"SHOULD I TRY THESE PMS GUMMIES?"

My sister is one of the many people in my life who regularly texts me before spending money on a wellness fad that seems too good to be true.

"Advil is cheaper and easier," I write back after doing the obligatory PubMed search on the ingredients listed on the product's website. (This kind of research comes free when you're related to me, but I'll teach you how to do it yourself in chapter 6.)

I checked the website she had texted me and saw that the ingredient label lists *Vitex agnus-castus,* a natural ingredient derived from a shrub commonly found in the Mediterranean, which limited research has actually shown to help some people with various PMS symptoms. That said, a 2017 systematic review of the research on this ingredient concluded that the effects "should be viewed as merely explorative and, at best, overestimating the real treatment effect."[20] Basically, we need more research to show if it's actually effective over placebos. It also has dong quai, a Chinese herb that is thought to help with PMS, although there is currently no quality clinical research in humans to confirm that.[21]

But here's the biggie: The research I found suggests that these ingredients could *also* affect your estrogen or dopamine levels, so they're not recommended for lots of people with certain conditions or those taking certain medications. Unfortunately, that's not stated in big bold letters on the website next to all the awesome claims—which haven't been evaluated by the FDA, naturally. I have to click around for a few minutes before I find a suggestion that says to talk to your doctor before taking it, especially if you have any conditions or are taking any medications (so, you know, most people).

Plus, at around $30 a bottle for a one-month supply, these gummies are much more expensive than taking an anti-inflammatory for a few days each month (the PMS plan that most of us have been resigned to).

I send a text-friendly version of all of this to my sister.

"Great point!" she texts back.

PMS is one of those things that we're often told is "normal," "no big deal," or "just part of the hand you've been dealt." But when you spend roughly 25 percent of every month (or more) dealing with excruciating cramps, holding your boobs when you go down the stairs, sporting large-and-in-charge pimples, and generally feeling shitty, tired, grumpy, and swollen, then you know that none of this feels "normal" or "no big deal." This sucks.

This monthly misery may be common and generally inconsequential by medical standards, but that certainly doesn't mean you have to suck it up and deal with it. And if medical innovation has figured out how to make robot-assisted surgery a thing, you would think that they would be able to dole out some solid PMS solutions, too. All of this is to say that I completely understand the allure of a product that claims to rid you of your PMS by eating a delicious gummy candy every day. Honestly, I've spent $30 on dumber stuff.

As a person with a period that typically comes in like a crampy, bitchy wrecking ball every month, I get the temptation. I would love to down some gummies and not experience PMS! But I also know from my job to do my own research on the ingredients before succumbing to a fantastic marketing strategy. Unfortunately, not everyone knows that's necessary—or even where to start—when presented with an adorable pastel product that promises to fix an annoying body problem. And I think that's why the wellness industry is so damn successful.

The wellness industry is reported to be a $4.5 trillion market, and I've had a front-row seat to watch its growth over the last decade. I'm basically their prime target—a young(ish) woman with disposable income, an interest in her health, and a whole lot of concerns about her body. If that sounds like you, too, then you've also probably had your social media feeds plastered with wellness products over the years.

Whether we're searching for it or not, we're constantly bombarded by the message that our bodies are broken and need fixing; that our health is suboptimal and could be so much better.

And, yeah, let's be honest, I've also been a wellness industry consumer many times, too. Sometimes that means trying the products that get sent to me unsolicited in hopes of editorial coverage. Other times it means entering my credit card information on some page I stumbled onto from Instagram, because look how many comments there are from people who say this product changed their life?!

But as the wellness market becomes more and more saturated with products aimed primarily at women, it seems it's only furthering our stress and confusion around what our bodies actually need to thrive.

Whether we're searching for it or not, we're constantly bombarded by the message that our bodies are broken and need fixing; that our health is suboptimal and could be so much better. And when the wellness cure of the moment doesn't make us feel any better, we're right back where we started at the beginning of the health-stress cycle, freaked out and insecure about our seemingly subpar bodies.

The unfortunate reality is that, for many people, it's a lot easier to just click "Buy" than it is to do a ton of research on every buzzy new health product that sounds fantastic. That's why I'm happy to drop whatever I'm up to and do some digging when someone asks me about a health trend. It's essentially the abbreviated version of what I did as a health editor.

But not everyone has my cell phone number and can text me when they come across something that claims to give them better skin, better sleep, better orgasms, better whatever. I guess I could just drop my number in here and cut this book short, but I'd rather help you learn how to finely tune your own wellness bullshit detector. And that starts with *just paying attention*.

What I really want you to take away from this chapter is a heightened awareness of the health messages you're getting all the damn time—whether it's in commercials, on Instagram, or even from that personal trainer at the gym who won't stop talking to you about the keto diet. (Bro, you're not a dietitian, please stop.)

The goal isn't to deter you from ever trying anything new or participating in wellness culture. The goal is to help you be a more conscious and informed consumer so that you don't get duped into wasting time, money, and energy on things you just don't need.

What is the wellness industry?

So let's talk about that big, thriving wellness industry. If that concept feels a little nebulous to you, just think about some of the health-adjacent products and services that you can't go a day without hearing about. I see them primarily falling into the following categories:

○ **ALL-NATURAL EVERYTHING:** Made without . . . *something!* Something you don't want in or around your body, even if you're not totally sure why. All-natural tampons, toilet paper, face wipes, butt wipes, moisturizers, cleansers, acne fighters, cold remedies, pain relievers, and so on. If there's a well-established, science-backed, safe, and effective solution out there, the industry is going to find a natural one that may or may not work as well—or at all—but will probably make you feel better because it's free of things—though most likely costs more.

○ **PERSONALIZED WELLNESS:** These products seem so much more legit than what you've been buying and using for years because they're formulated *just for you*. Or, at least, it seems that way because you took a really long quiz and got some product recommendations that seem pretty personalized. I'm talking about things like made-for-you vitamins, supplements, skin care, hair care, protein powder, etc.

○ **DIY HEALTH:** This is anything that claims to diagnose or treat something that should really be diagnosed and treated in a medical setting—whether it's problems with your skin, gut, period, sexual health, vaginal health, or pretty much anything else that you'd really prefer to deal with at home, thank you very much. The accuracy, efficacy, and usefulness of things like these vary, of course, but the one thing they all have in common is a warning that you should probably see a real medical professional at some point.

○ **THE INGREDIENT DU JOUR:** OMG have you heard about CBD? Alkaline water? Activated charcoal? Turmeric? Apple cider vinegar? Ginger? Green coffee bean extract? Probiotics? Who knows what launches these things into the zeitgeist with such force that everyone from your boss to your hairdresser to your great aunt is suddenly talking about it. (JK, we all know it's Facebook. It's always Facebook.) These are typically things that have always existed and always done . . . *something*. But when the wellness industry gets ahold of them, that's when you start seeing them as special ingredients in everything from smoothies to skin care products. Does it belong there? Is it doing anything? Who knows? But it's there!

Of course, these examples aren't the only extensions of the wellness industry. Wellness culture goes far beyond that, including things like health clubs, boutique fitness classes, wellness retreats, weight loss programs, wearable health tech, and much more.

When I try to define the wellness industry for someone, I say that it's essentially the **commercialization of wellness.** It's anything that makes money off of you taking care of yourself outside of a conventional health setting. It's mostly concerned with fixing problems, rather than preventing them. It promotes wellness as a thing that you do—in consistent and often costly ways—rather than a state of being. Taking part in it is like a badge of honor, signaling to others that you're someone who gives a damn about their health. Maybe that's why it feels so good to buy and try these things, even if we aren't always sure if or when or how they'll work.

There's big business in telling someone that their body or their health could be better. And, in general, we're pretty easy to convince when we're already so tired, stressed out, and unfamiliar with what's happening in or on our bodies. No one can fault you for wanting to feel better. We all want to feel better!

And that's where the wellness industry comes barging in like a nosy, inappropriate, boundaryless friend. "Hi! Oh, wow have you gained weight? You should try Whole30. And, honey, your hair is looking a little meh. Have you heard about biotin supplements? How's your poop by the way? Did I tell you about these probiotics I got from my health coach? She's changed my life—and my skin thanks to her own line of all-natural CBD skin care. You should come with me to her seven-day wellness retreat. It's transformative. You look really tired."

That's exhausting, right? You would not want to be friends with that friend! But we put up with her because occasionally she's fun and entertaining and means well and honestly once she gave you a night cream that didn't suck, so maybe she knows what she's talking about sometimes?

> *If you remember one thing from this chapter, let it be this: The wellness industry is trying to sell you something.*

To me, that's what the wellness industry is like: a friend with an endless supply of health tips, tricks, and recommendations—some of which are bull-shit, some of which are legit, all of which will cost you money.

If you remember one thing from this chapter, let it be this: The wellness industry is trying to sell you something.

Now, that doesn't have to be as scary as it sounds. It's just a reality. The guy who owns the produce stand two blocks from my apartment is trying to sell me something, too, and that doesn't make him a manipulative, malicious person. And I'm not saying the wellness industry is inherently bad, either. I mean, it's an industry predicated on helping you take care of yourself, so the intentions (I'd like to think, at least) are good. But at the end of the day these are businesses trying to make a buck, and it's important to keep that in mind.

Also, hi, I am part of the wellness industry. I've been writing health content—mostly for wellness brands—for the past decade. I, too, have profited off of telling people how to take care of themselves. I've also spent a lot of that money back on the wellness industry. I've paid a ridiculous amount of it on fitness classes in New York City. I have ongoing subscriptions for organic smoothies, pastel razors, and nutritious meal kits. I once sat uncomfortably perched on a pillow during a sound bath (not for me!). I have a meditation app on my phone that I use a ton. I pay an annual membership for access to a bougie primary care practice that boasts no wait times and 24/7 telehealth

> **It's your money,**
> **your time,**
> **your choice.**

services. I gulp down some Emergen-C every time I feel a tickle in my throat.

I guess what I'm trying to say is that you're allowed to have a personal care arsenal that includes things that aren't all science-backed or medically necessary. You're allowed to engage with the wellness industry in whatever ways make you feel good. It's your money, your time, your choice.

But here's the thing: Not everyone has the money or the time to spend on wellness products that don't actually make you well. And that's why I want these wellness companies—these wellness messages—to do better. According to the CDC, 6 out of 10 U.S. adults live with at least one chronic condition.[22] When we're desperate for solutions that help us regain our lives, we don't have time for snake oil and pseudoscience.

WHAT TWITTER'S FAVORITE DOCTOR THINKS ABOUT THE WELLNESS INDUSTRY

"To me, wellness is very predatory," says Jen Gunter, MD.

In case you aren't one of Gunter's more than 331,000 Twitter followers, allow me to introduce you to one of my favorite wellness industry watch-dogs. Gunter is board-certified in obstetrics and gynecology as well as in pain medicine. A 2016 profile in *The Cut* named her "Twitter's resident gynecologist." But what I've always appreciated most about Gunter is her very low tolerance for wellness bullshit and the people profiting from it.

I knew I could count on her for fascinating insights into why we're some-times so much more interested in wellness fads than we are in going to the doctor. Why do so many people shun antibiotics and annual physicals while shelling out for unproven supplements and IV wellness infusions?

"It's an amazing, amazing phenomenon of branding isn't it?" Gunter says of the wellness industry. "They are offering what I would say is the worst part of medicine: expensive therapies that don't work, pills that you don't need that are potentially harmful, and unindicated lab tests. But what they are giving people in many ways is *trying* and *validation*. So that's why I think it's important to look to that industry and say: *Well, what are they offering that people are clearly missing?*"

The answer, it seems, isn't just fast fixes, but also compassion and empathy. Maybe that's where the wellness industry found its footing. Maybe that's why it's so damn tempting.

"If you're not being listened to and you have symptoms, where are you gonna go? You're gonna go where people are listening to you. I absolutely understand that," remarks Gunter. "So I think we just have to look at *why* people haven't been listened to and how all the messaging sort of preys on that."

The wellness industry knows you better than you think.

It's no coincidence that the wellness industry has thrived alongside a growing distrust and discontent with traditional medical care. In my eyes, the wellness industry is answering a call to action from frustrated, fed-up patients everywhere: we want solutions, but we also want someone to listen. And I know there are responsible innovators and brands answering that call. But there are also far too many companies that are using this vulnerability as an invitation to sell you something that is at best a waste of your money and at worst actually harmful.

I'm going to let you in on a few fundamental truths that the wellness industry already knows about you. I know they know this because I spent the better part of my career as part of the wellness industry, and I knew it, too. I kept these fundamental truths in mind whenever I created content to help people take better care of themselves. But I also try to keep them in mind whenever I'm the person consuming the health content—usually just as stressed out about my body as you are.

I want you to know what the wellness industry knows, because that will help you pinpoint the intention behind those health messages you're getting all the time. That way, you can better decide if this is something you want to actually engage with—or if this message seems to be relying more on your insecurities and your desires than it is on actual proven benefits.

Here are five fundamental truths that the wellness industry knows about you:

1 We all have issues with our bodies and our health that we'd like to address.

2 We tend to want solutions that are simple, convenient, and discreet.

3 We all have various spheres of influence that impact our decision-making.

4 For so many of us, traditional health care is unaffordable and inaccessible.

5 For others, investing in our health is something we're happy to splurge on.

When you keep those truths in mind, it's not hard to see how people and brands can use that information to sell you something. Who needs proven benefits or FDA approval when you have these tactics? Here are just a few examples:

○ **They can mine your health issues and insecurities to offer you solutions with big claims and no actual science behind them.**

- They can offer you a product or service that's undeniably easier than going to the doctor—even if you'll most likely have to see a doctor for this issue eventually anyway.

- They can tailor their message or create their whole distribution model based on who you tend to listen to, whether that's your Facebook friends, your favorite celebrities, or your go-to health magazine.

- They can position themselves as the antidote to the confusing, frustrating, expensive-as-hell health care system that nobody likes anyway.

- They can also position themselves as a worthy investment in your health— something you'd be wise to spend your money on.

My best piece of advice for dealing with the wellness industry is this: have a healthy dose of skepticism. Keep in mind that, at the end of the day, the wellness industry is trying to sell you something. It's a moneymaking industry, and it's thriving because we're all so damn anxious about our bodies all the time for a multitude of reasons, not least of which is what it means to be deemed "less than" in our society—whether that means having a disability, a chronic illness, acne, or simply less energy and youthfulness than you once had. I'm pretty sure we all have things about our bodies that we want to change or improve. That's part of having a body. Just be mindful of the solutions that you spend your time, money, and energy on.

My inbox, a horror story

I'm going to be honest, my inbox scares the hell out of me sometimes. I'm primarily talking about my old work inbox when I was a full-time health editor, but even now I still sometimes hear from a particularly determined publicist.

The emails and press releases I get can be incredibly triggering for someone with health anxiety, particularly if I'm already feeling stressed about a specific symptom (like this headache I've had basically all week) and then I get a bunch of emails with subject lines like this:

- Your Morning Headache Might Be a Sign of This

- Re: Migraine Awareness Month—Want to speak to a neurologist?

- Relieve Tension Headaches Naturally with This New Product

- You Might Have This Toxic Ticking Bomb in Your Body

(Before you assume I'm exaggerating, I want to assure you that I only changed two or three words in those subject lines. That's really just a small sampling of what I was faced with every day when I opened my email.)

As triggering as that could be, it was also fascinating: It was basically a sneak peak of the health trends that everyone was about to see out in the wild. I was getting pitch emails about the same products that I would soon find in ads plastered on the subway, in sponsored posts on Instagram, and in group texts with friends who ask, "Has anyone ever tried this? Do I need this?"

It's pretty wild when I stop to think about it. My inbox was essentially a bird's-eye view of the wellness messages that we're all getting exposed to every single day. And most of this messaging serves one of two purposes: to offer up solutions for a health problem you're currently stressing about or to give you a new health problem to stress about (so they can solve it, obviously).

Of course, I also got emails containing genuinely interesting new research or helpful experts to connect with. But, overwhelmingly, it was like the wellness industry threw up directly into my inbox.

On average, I probably got around 15 emails per day about new wellness trends, products, and services. It was a lot of detoxes, supplements, organic alternatives, or pricey procedures. According to these emails, you're not actually the best version of yourself until you're in ketosis, rejuvenating your vagina, and putting CBD in every single one of your orifices.

I spent almost 10 years dutifully digging into the research on whatever wellness fad was currently trending and more often than not debunking most of the major claims. I did the legwork to tell you why your vagina doesn't need jade eggs, vaginal steams, lasers, douches, or yogurt. I assigned stories all about the science or lack thereof behind celery juice, raw water, and CBD skin care. And, honestly, you start to feel like a real buzzkill. Listen, I want celery water to cure IBS just as much as the next person, but it just doesn't.

The companies that sell these products seem to rely on the fact that you don't know a whole lot about the science on these issues, that you tend to turn to the internet for answers, and that you'll probably just go ahead and buy it before you look into the research or ask your doctor.

The ads often feel more like a battle cry than a commercial, with a message that mixes mainstream feminist sensibilities and fearmongering.

○ *We actually care about women.* (Translation: We know you've probably had a doctor tell you it's just stress.)

○ *You deserve to know what you're putting in your body.* (Translation: Those other companies aren't being transparent with you.)

○ *We use science to make you feel better.* (Translation: You should trust us because we mentioned science.)

Over the years, I became almost totally desensitized to this endless avalanche of wellness pitches. Most days I just hit Select All > Mark As Read a few times so the big bold letters weren't taunting me from my inbox.

But a weird thing happened whenever I went on vacation—completely removed from my office and from Work Casey. I'd check my email from my towel on a beach somewhere—a habit I swear I'll break one of these days—and I'd catch one of those familiar subject lines, except in this situation it wouldn't seem so familiar. It would be jarring and unexpected, sometimes a little absurd, and other times even . . . intriguing? I'd click on it and start reading about some new survey or fad, my health editor defenses temporarily deactivated while out of office. And the message—whatever it was—hit differently.

I *am* bloated and gassy! I *would* like to say goodbye to tummy troubles. Wait . . . do I need this supplement? Should I ask for a sample?

Then, eventually, my years of health reporting experience would kick in and I'd suddenly read the email as an editor again—quickly combing through it for any mention of FDA approval, peer-reviewed research, or even an actual medical doctor endorsement. When I didn't find it, it got marked as read with the others.

But that weird vacation brain moment tells me so much about the disconnect between me and my readers. I spend basically all day, every day thinking and talking and writing about health concepts that most people very rarely spend any energy on. Because of that, I often wrongly assume that everyone has the same context that I do—which, of course, they don't! Maybe you've spent the last 10 years studying law, becoming an architect, building a family, traveling the Middle East, or something else that is very unlike spending a decade covering the health industry.

So, of course, the same message would hit you differently than it would me. When you hear about a new wellness trend, you're receiving that information as someone who has lived a different life with different priorities and different knowledge. I can't assume that we all would see that same pitch and think, *Wow, what a waste of money/what an offensive implication about our bodies/what a load of shit.*

Our lives, our needs, our circumstances all influence what we pay attention to, what we believe, and what we choose to spend our time, money, and energy on. Just like we don't all have the same bodies and body concerns, we don't all have the same resources to spend taking care of them.

And that's why I get so worked up about the seemingly silly, harmless wellness trends: they aren't so silly or harmless for everyone.

Can I live?!

I know I sound like a serious downer right now. Why can't I just let you chug your celery juice in peace?! So let me better explain my stance on wellness trends: Wellness trends can sometimes be harmless, delightful, and enriching—even if there is zero science whatsoever behind them. But wellness trends become *harmful* when they put your health at risk, by either directly causing harm or delaying you from seeking treatment.

Let's take celery juice as an example: Chugging it first thing in the morning isn't going to directly hurt you, but if you're doing that instead of taking medication for your high blood pressure, that can have serious consequences. Similarly, splurging on organic cotton tampons isn't going to harm your vagina, but if you're doing it because you think it'll get rid of that vaginal itch you're experiencing—rather than going to a doctor to diagnose that vaginal itch—then we've got a problem.

The key here is realizing that it's not just the ingredients in health products that can be harmful, but also the messaging that surrounds them if it leads you to believe that you can manage symptoms on your own when you need a professional. And for someone like me, with a strong urge to avoid medical care, this kind of marketing can be incredibly tempting. It's simultaneously preying on your anxieties and giving you permission to *not* seek medical care for that thing you're worried about. It's keeping you trapped in the health-stress cycle even longer.

This is my biggest gripe with so many of those vaginal hygiene products. The marketing is all about empowering you to take care of your vaginal health, banish odor, kick yeast infections to the curb, and just generally make your vagina sparkle and shine. (Okay maybe they don't actually say that last part . . . but they might.) Here's the problem: If you're experiencing a vaginal odor that is out of the ordinary for you or if you think you're having yeast infection after yeast infection, you need to bring that shit up with a medical professional—not drop $50 on vagina wipes, washes, and suppositories.

> *We have limited resources when it comes to taking care of ourselves—whether we're talking about the money, time, or effort that we're willing to spend on it—so you want to make sure that you're using those resources wisely.*

We have limited resources when it comes to taking care of ourselves—whether we're talking about the money, time, or effort that we're willing to spend on it—so you want to make sure that you're using those resources wisely.

Take Sarah, for instance. Sarah is a 33-year-old mom who works at a service job without health care benefits. She's been dealing with symptoms of depression and anxiety for over a year, and every day she feels like her fuse is getting shorter, her patience is wearing thinner, she's on the verge of tears all the time. She feels like she's treading water constantly and the shore seems so far away. Sarah knows that she needs to take care of her mental health, but she doesn't know how. She doesn't have money to spend seeing a therapist or a doctor—let alone for the childcare she'd need to coordinate so that she could get out of the house for a while. Even teletherapy options cost money. But also, she doesn't need a therapist—she's not "crazy," and she grew up hearing that only "crazy" people go to therapy.

Then Sarah sees an ad for a product on Facebook that promises to boost energy, mental clarity, and mood. The ad says it can help with anxiety, depression, and mood swings. It says it's a natural, science-backed remedy, which makes her feel better. It's pricey at $75 a bottle, which probably means it's worth it. Plus, if it works, that onetime price is cheaper than any of the other options she has. She's never heard of the ingredients before, but it all sounds legit. And think about it: In an ideal world, she'd just take this discreetly and feel better. No one would ever have to know that she was struggling so hard that she bought something off the internet. She gets it, thinking, *What the hell? I just need to feel better. What's the harm?*

I'll tell you the harm. In an unlikely but worst-case scenario, this supplement contains something that could put her health at risk. Maybe it doesn't mix well with something else she's taking—whether that's over-the-counter medicines or prescriptions or even food and alcohol. And because she doesn't have health insurance, she probably isn't consulting her doctor about all of this before she takes it. I don't know what's really in this supplement any more than Sarah does, so really, who knows what could happen?

In a much more likely scenario, nothing happens—good or bad. Sarah is out $75 plus shipping and handling. It's been a month and she's no closer to feeling any relief from the depression and anxiety that is enveloping her every single day. The only difference between her now and her a month ago is that she's now lost both money and time that she can't get back—money and time that she really hoped would make her feel like herself again. She's still frustrated, confused, and scared. But now she's angry with herself, too. How did she fall for something like this?

(I realize that there's also a best-case scenario here, too. One in which Sarah feels better and the internet supplement actually cured her anxiety and depression. I would love for that to be the case. But I'm also a pragmatist as well as someone who has been writing about mental health for a long time. That magical supplement doesn't exist. Or if it does, it's just an antidepressant being doled out without medical supervision.)

Scenarios like this are why I want us all to be aware of the messaging coming at us from all angles. Sure, most of it is harmless. Sure, some of it might be genuinely useful or at the very least give you a pleasant placebo effect when you use it. But all of that hinges on you having money, time, and effort to spare on these little experiments. Many people don't have that luxury. They just want to feel better, often because traditional medical care is unaffordable, inaccessible, or historically unreliable for them.

The message matters.

I know I said that the wellness industry is mainly focused on fixing problems, but it can also create new problems—or at least turn our attention to something that we never even knew was a problem before. When so much of the messaging is around how to fix problems with your body, there will inevitably be times when you'll be inundated with solutions for issues you didn't even know you had but now are acutely aware of—especially if you deal with health anxiety the way I do.

How many times have you seen an ad for some wellness product and thought: *Oh, wow, do I need that?* It happens to me all the time. I'll see a headline about 11 Ways to Deal with Thinning Hair in Your Thirties and become hyperfocused on my hairline for the next several months. (*Is it thinning? OMG yes, what is that little patch over there? IS THAT MY SKULL?*) I'll see an ad for teeth whiteners and suddenly become incredibly aware of the color of my teeth. (*Did I just not look at my teeth for the last 10 years? When did they become this color?!*)

The messages we're getting about our bodies—even in ads on TV or Facebook—can absolutely change the way we think and feel about them.

They can make us more critical, more anxious, more concerned with finding "solutions."

Gunter pointed out a particularly salient theme that she sees often—much more often than is medically warranted: "This idea that your vagina is one step away from absolute mayhem. Almost every women's magazine has something about pubic hair, vaginas, or vulvas every time. It's amazing to me. That sort of reinforces that you're constantly broken."

Think about all those infomercials for ways to deal with "unsightly" cellulite, "embarrassing" stretch marks, and "disgusting" pores. Now let's all take a second to remember that all of those things are simply just features of a human body. There is nothing inherently pathological about any of them. But we've been told that, aesthetically, they are problems that need to be fixed. Of course, because these are just features of a body, any at-home attempts at fixing them aren't likely to do anything. You're going to need something a little stronger (read: lasers) to remove something that has every right to be on your body.

Oh, and can we talk about the fact that the ads for these solutions feature primarily—if not exclusively—women? It's never a dude slathering on something to rid him of his cellulite, stretch marks, or pores—even though men can also have all three. It's always a woman. This is something that, once you think about it, you won't be able to stop noticing examples of.

How often do we see ads for products that will make penises smell better? How often do we see men featured in commercials for antiaging skin care? How often are men told to shove a jade egg up one of their orifices? The answer to all three is, of course, almost never.

Now, I know that men aren't completely spared by the wellness industry—they're just targeted in different ways, primarily with products aimed at giving them more hair, more muscles, more sex drive, more stamina. They're similarly told to address basic issues of human variation.

And then, of course, there's the one section of the wellness industry that targets all of us: diet and weight loss products. In this case, they're all advertised to everyone with a slight variation on the same message: You can't possibly be happy, healthy, or really truly living your best life unless you're thin. But, you know, not too thin.

These ads and the products within them aren't going anywhere anytime soon. I can't shield you from them, nor would I want to, because it's totally your prerogative to put whatever you want in and on your body to make yourself feel better or more confident. But hopefully, by being more aware of these messages, you can start to notice their implications, question them, roll your eyes at them, and maybe even sometimes tell them to kindly fuck off.

Let's stop trying to make health trendy.

When it comes to taking care of our health, we all want a quick and easy fix. But it's not just that. We also seem to want fixes that have a little bit of an edge to them. We want trendy new hacks that are surprising and cool. Or we want old, ancient remedies repackaged in an Instagram-friendly way. We want them to be backed up by science, but not necessarily so mainstream that they're FDA approved. We want our health solutions to be interesting, cute, counterintuitive, and unconventional. But we also want them to work.

The well-established wellness wisdom—eat fruits and vegetables, get enough sleep, stay active, you know the drill—just isn't sexy. It also isn't accessible or realistic for a huge number of folks. So we reject, ignore, or conveniently forget these trusted tips and go searching for some kind of hack instead.

I do it, too, I swear. More than once I've felt like garbage after spending the better part of the weekend eating cheese doodles in the prone position on the couch, then stumbled upon an ad for probiotics and thought, *Yes, that's totally what I need to boost my gut health.* No bitch, you need broccoli and a walk.

We love to think that this new simple, sexy, surprising supplement is going to be the key to better health, when in reality, there is tons of research-backed advice for better health out there. We just don't find it as interesting or attainable.

> *The truth is, health isn't trendy. And anyone who says otherwise is probably trying to sell you something.*

There's an ad I see online all the time that I cannot stand—I'm sure you've seen it, too—that perfectly sums up this ridiculousness. The ad says something to the effect of "Doctors Don't Want You to Know About This Miracle Cure!" (It's usually paired with a stock image of a common body concern, like wrinkles or dark circles or varicose veins.)

You guys. I know a lot of doctors. I promise you that if there were miracle cures, they would want you to know about them. They would love to charge you a copay to tell you about them and send you on your way. Pharmaceutical companies would love it, too. Ditto for the FDA.

Don't you think that if there were actually a miracle cure it would be getting real airtime and not be buried in a weird ad at the bottom of an article? These ads persist not because they're selling anything legit but because people click on them.

We're always looking for the next best health thing. We're encouraged by the wellness industry to never be satisfied with our bodies the way they currently exist or are currently being cared for. We're convinced that there's a secret solution out there somewhere that we just haven't found or tried yet.

Is this a tendency people have always had? Or is it something that's both a function of the wellness industry and a way to fuel that industry? My guess is that it's the latter. Either way, it's a tendency that we need to pay attention to and analyze if we want to make more informed decisions about our health.

The truth is, health isn't trendy. And anyone who says otherwise is probably trying to sell you something.

PART II

BOOSTING YOUR HEALTH LITERACY, YOUR WELLNESS BULLSHIT DETECTOR, AND YOUR CARE TOOLKIT

ow that we've covered why we tend to stress and panic about our health, it's time to learn how to stop that spiral. Here's the good news: You're basically halfway there. You already have a better understanding of why we're so often stressed about our bodies and why our quest for answers usually leaves us even more confused. But knowledge is just half the equation.

Consider my situation, way back in the introduction: I was a health editor who had written several articles explaining that an abnormal Pap smear is typically no big deal. And still, when I got that phone call from my doctor, my first thought was *Great I'm dying and infertile and probably have cancer.*

Consider another one of my not-so-proud moments: I was a health editor whose beat was reproductive health—I could tell you the efficacy rates of each birth control method off the top of my head—but after a condom broke during casual sex, I insisted on taking Plan B . . . even though I was already taking the birth control pill (you know, Plan A). Because . . . well . . . who's to say I didn't maybe miss one pill that month or something? Really, honestly, *WHO CAN BE SURE?!*

Or what about all the times that I toss back a handful of vitamins whenever I feel even a hint of a scratch in my throat, even though I've written and edited countless articles about the lack of definitive research showing that does anything.

What I've learned from nearly a decade of health reporting and a lifetime of being anxious about my body is this: When it comes to worrying about your health, it sometimes doesn't matter what the doctors say, what the studies say, or what the headlines say; it can be really easy to get swept up in your own fear and uncertainty—no matter how much information you're armed with. It's why we're often willing to try anything when we're struggling—lack of peer-reviewed research and all of your better judgment be damned.

That's why the following chapters aren't an exhaustive list of what's legit and what's bullshit in the current wellness zeitgeist. Sure, that would be fun to read—and you can probably find that online, for what it's worth—but it wouldn't necessarily help you to think critically long term about all the health messages you'll be exposed to in the future and the way that you'll think about your health on a day-to-day basis.

Instead, I want to arm you with strategies and techniques that will boost your health literacy. I want you to feel empowered to do your own research and to be your own advocate. I want you to confidently call bullshit on a wellness hack that asks for your time and money without any clinical research to back it up. I want you to know that the next time you notice a weird symptom or hear some very concerning health news, you have the same resources at your disposal as I do.

So let's get into it.

How to listen to your body just enough

WE'RE TOLD ALL THE TIME TO LISTEN TO OUR BODIES. To be mindful of our breathing. To tune into what's happening. And don't get me wrong, that's all incredibly valuable stuff. But this is also true: sometimes your body is noisy as hell for no good reason. Mine, for instance, likes to pull the fire alarm for shits and giggles all the time.

If you can relate, then you see why it's not always as simple as listening to your body and reporting back. For some of us, there's a fine line between listening to our bodies and becoming hypervigilant about our bodies.

I have no problem listening to my body. I do, however, have a problem tuning that bitch out sometimes.

There are moments when I can't hear anything but my body. I'll be laying on the couch, watching *The Office* for the four millionth time, and I'm suddenly hyperaware of my heartbeat or a feeling in my stomach or a pain in my left boob or a tremor in my hand. Honestly anything.

> *For some of us, there's a fine line between listening to our bodies and becoming hyper-vigilant about our bodies.*

It's probably nothing, says the health editor side of my brain, who knows that I have maybe one risk factor for that thing I'm freaking out about.

Okay, but it also could be something, says the anxious side of my brain, who is significantly louder and harder to ignore.

I am very often hypervigilant about my body. And I'm sure being a health editor who was constantly reading and writing about health issues didn't help the matter.

I'll never forget the time a coworker said to me: "It must be so nice to have all that medical knowledge on the top of your head from all the reporting you've done." Spoiler alert: It is not!

I know that I'm very fortunate to have access to all of this information. I don't take for granted the fact that my education, experience, and opportunity allows me to chat with experts at the CDC, the Mayo Clinic, and Johns Hopkins—to name-drop a few of my favorite sources. But the truth is that sometimes the more information I have, the more I have to get anxious about. It's like having a lot of meaningless trivia floating around in your head— except the trivia is themed "Stuff You Might Die From." When I read about the symptoms of various illnesses, that shit stays with me. And when I feel a hint of one, my mind immediately goes to that illness. (Case in point: fried rice syndrome!)

It's possible that this is true for you, too, on some level. After all, we all have truly unprecedented access to health content these days. You can't watch the news without hearing a bunch of scary health headlines. You can't turn on *Grey's Anatomy* without finding out about a rare condition that can kill off a charming new character within an episode. You can't go on social media without seeing someone share their story of a freckle that was actually stage III melanoma.

Maybe none of this bothers you. If that's the case: wow, what a carefree life you must live! But for the rest of us, all that nightmare fuel can make "listening to your body" really fucking scary.

Maybe you've only dealt with this occasionally—like while in the middle of a deadly pandemic, possibly? I know I'm not the only one who became hyperfocused on every little symptom I experienced as soon as the COVID-19 pandemic began.

Is that regular shortness of breath or coronavirus-related shortness of breath? Have I always gotten this winded after 10 push-ups, or can I just not remember the last time I actually did 10 push-ups? Is that a fever or am I just hot from all these push-ups?

My point is, "listening to your body" is not a diagnostic tool for a reason. It's important, without a doubt, but it can also be a deeply flawed and fraught practice. For many of us, listening to our bodies can quickly become a game of Is That Supposed to Happen or Am I Dying?

Let me share just a small sampling of random body things that I've absolutely lost my shit over—and, by that, I mean that I became preoccupied with this symptom for . . . longer than I'd care to admit: the amount of hair I was shedding on a regular basis, the amount of times I peed during the day, how much my eyes were watering, some occasional boob pain, various patches of dry skin, so many different kinds of stomach pains, jaw pain, eye floaters, back pain, suspicious nail ridges, head pain, various rashes, dizziness, tiredness, the smell/consistency/frequency of my discharge, the way I was breathing, and so so much more, but I'm going to stop there because I did say this was going to be a *small* sampling.

Now, some people might notice any of those and think, *huh, that's weird.* And then they go on living their lives. I am not one of those people. And, if you're reading this book, chances are you aren't one of those people either.

What the princess and the pea has to do with health anxiety

So why do some of us become so panicked and preoccupied at every little symptom, while others are barely bothered? To answer that, I called board-certified psychologist Jenny Yip, PsyD. Yip is a nationally recognized expert on OCD and anxiety disorders, and she knows what it's like to live with anxiety, having experienced OCD herself.

Yip explains that some people just have a lower threshold for bodily discomfort, which may explain why some of us have this heightened body awareness that causes so much anxiety while others barely register those little changes.

"It's all on a continuum of those who are constantly checking their body, constantly looking for symptoms, and those who will be a little bit more moderate," says Yip.

Hypervigilance about what's happening in our bodies is common—it might be something you deal with occasionally (like when there's a global pandemic) or pretty much all the time (hi, it's me). But if this preoccupation with specific symptoms becomes excessive and causes you significant distress, you might even meet the criteria for somatic symptom disorder.

In the introduction, I briefly went over those two main conditions in the DSM-5 that relate to health anxiety: somatic symptom disorder and illness anxiety disorder. (See page 14.) As I mentioned, there's a lot of overlap between the two. And, crucially, it's possible to experience facets of these disorders without meeting the clinical criteria for either of them. But when it comes to focusing excessively on specific symptoms—that's a pretty classic feature of somatic symptom disorder. (FYI: Having somatic symptom disorder doesn't mean that the symptoms aren't real—some people with somatic symptom disorder know exactly what's causing their symptoms—but a diagnosis means that the focus on your symptoms is excessive, it's causing you a lot of anxiety, and you're spending so much time and energy worrying about these symptoms that it's interfering with your life.)

"We all have a different pain threshold or discomfort threshold," explains Yip. "And for people with somatic symptom disorder, their pain or discomfort threshold may be lower. And therefore they aren't able to tolerate their bodily discomfort the same way that someone else with a higher threshold may be able to tolerate. They're more sensitive to bodily discomfort, their threshold for the discomfort is lower, and they are constantly hypervigilant about their body."

Take, for instance, your heartbeat. Most people don't pay much attention to it, only really tuning in when they notice it pounding in their chests after a brutal workout or before a stressful presentation. Otherwise, you probably don't think about your heartbeat all that much. But for some of us (*raises hand*) you might pay attention to your mundane bodily functions way more than that, and not because you want to, but because you're highly sensitive to any slight discomfort in your body.

When I was little, my mom used to refer to me as the princess and the pea. You know, that weird fairy tale where a prince and his overbearing queen mom make a woman sleep on a bed of 20 mattresses to see if she can feel the pea underneath it all, assuming that only that could determine if she was a real princess? Yeah, it makes no sense, but when I was a little girl, I did take solace in the fact that I must be part princess if I was so freaking sensitive that I could feel even the slightest issue. It could be a fold in my sock, a tag touching me, or even a shirt with the audacity to have a turtleneck—I couldn't stand it. As an adult, I'm not that high maintenance anymore, but I am still hypervigilant about any symptom, any discomfort, any small change in my body's baseline.

Now, I've never been formally diagnosed with somatic symptom disorder, but I can rattle off more than a few instances in my life when I was consumed by panic and anxiety around specific symptoms, and it absolutely interfered with my life.

I was listening to my body alright. I was listening so intently that I could barely hear anything else.

It's hard to describe what it feels like to live in this near-constant state of anxiety around your health, but the best thing I can compare it to is when you were a kid and you knew you had done something wrong and it was only a matter of time before you'd get caught. You know that pit in your stomach that crops up when you realize that you're going to be found out and there's *nothing you can do about it*? You can't fully focus on anything else, can't enjoy anything else, because it's always there in the back of your mind? That's what health anxiety feels like to me.

It feels like you're going about your day, paying attention in meetings, laughing with your friends, being charming on a date, all the usual stuff—but just below the surface your mind is like, *Hey, remember that weird pain you felt earlier? It's probably cancer. K thanks, carry on!*

Yip has another metaphor she likes to use for anxiety: "It's like having a nightmare that keeps replaying in your mind like a broken record that you cannot wake up from. But nobody else can see your nightmare. And because your nightmare might be so irrational, so silly, so excessive, you might feel embarrassed for even disclosing this nightmare. And therefore you keep it to yourself. And it becomes a silent disease."

I have no idea if the people closest to me ever knew what I was going through during those moments of my life. I don't know why they would have. I put on a brave face. I went to parties and talked to my friends and appeared completely fine, but on the inside I was focused on this alternate reality that I had drummed up for myself based on my perceived symptoms: I'm actually pregnant. Or I actually have a life-altering chronic illness. Or I actually have a terminal illness that's quietly killing me. Or or or . . .

It took me a long time—too long—to realize that I wasn't pregnant or dying . . . I was still just the princess and the pea. Only the pea wasn't in my shoe or under my mattress—it was in my body. I probably would have reached this conclusion much faster had I reached out for help earlier. So let this be a reminder that if any of this is resonating with you, please don't be afraid to talk to someone about it. I wish I had sooner. Maybe then I would have realized that the nagging feeling that something was terribly wrong with my body was actually anxiety—not intuition.

But that's the tricky part of intuition, of feeling it in your bones. You might be feeling something, alright—in fact, I 100% believe you are—but that doesn't mean it's always something that needs to keep you up at night.

If you don't want to take it from me, maybe you'll appreciate this reminder from Abramowitz: "I'd like to point out to people that have health anxiety that it's not all in their head. They've been told often by physicians, 'Oh it's nothing; it's all in your head; whatever.' It's not. It's in their body. They're not making it up. But usually, the problem is that it's not as catastrophic as the person thinks. Often the tendency is to think hurt equals harm, or that if I notice something in my body—any little sensation— then it means I'm not healthy. And, of course, that's not true. Healthy bodies do all sorts of weird stuff."

> But that's the tricky part of intuition, of feeling it in your bones. You might be feeling something, alright— in fact, I 100% believe you are—but that doesn't mean it's always something that needs to keep you up at night.

That said, I realize that it's absolutely infuriating to hear that what you're freaking out about is actually no big deal and you just need to stop thinking about it. For starters, I have no way of knowing if what you're going through is actually a big deal or not. Even if I did, saying "just relax—it's probably nothing" is deeply unhelpful, because it negates a person's experience and minimizes their reality. There's a reason that "just relax" doesn't do shit for medical ailments *or* health anxiety.

So I'm not going to do that. Instead, I'm going to give you a few tips for listening to your body in a way that is compassionate, curious, and ideally a little less anxiety-provoking. Hopefully, they help you, too.

5 helpful tips for listening to your body

RESPECT THE MIND-BODY CONNECTION.

I promise, I am not going to tell you that anything is all in your head. What I *am* going to say is that what goes on in your head is often more important to your physical health than you might realize.

There is an enormous amount of research supporting a mind-body connection. Take, for instance, the role of stress in so many conditions. Stress is associated with a higher risk of respiratory viruses,[23] ulcers, [24] heart disease,[25] and type 2 diabetes.[26] And that's just the short list. Stress may also lead to flare-ups or more miserable symptoms in people who have certain conditions, like irritable bowel syndrome,[27] ulcerative colitis,[28] migraines,[29] multiple sclerosis,[30] and many others. When this happens, a doctor might say that stress is "exacerbating" your condition, which means that it's making it worse.

Chronic stress is even thought to be a crucial factor behind the disproportionate rates of illness and death in Black people. The term for this is *weathering*.[31] Weathering was first coined by Arline Geronimus, ScD, professor at the University of Michigan School of Public Health, whose research examines the role that the chronic stress of racism has on biological markers of aging and other health outcomes. Weathering is just one explanation for why Black people die from chronic conditions at a higher rate than others—like heart disease, type 2 diabetes, and cancer—conditions that have proven ties to chronic stress.

You wouldn't (or shouldn't) tell someone that their type 2 diabetes or multiple sclerosis is "all in their head"—we know that's not true—but your psychological health does play a role in these illnesses and many others.

The truth is that your mind and body are intimately connected, and yet sometimes it seems like we only extol the powers of our mental health when it's convenient. When we're looking for answers to our physical concerns, we rarely consider the role of our mental health. And I understand why: because we want something tangible and external to blame for our suffering and we want something concrete and easy to fix it. We don't want to hear that what's going on in our own heads could be playing a role—even if it's just a small, supporting role. We don't want to hear that the call is coming from inside the house.

Here's an example: A patient goes to the doctor with horrible stomach pains. It feels so bad, they assume their appendix must have burst, but it's also on fire and also maybe they're dying. It's that bad. The doctor does some poking around ("Does this hurt? How about here? What about when I do this?"), and asks the patient a few questions that seem relevant ("Any changes to your bowel movements? What about your diet? Any other symptoms—fever, bleeding, bloating, etc.?"). But then the doctor hits the patient with this one: "Have you been under a lot of stress lately?"

Really, doc? REALLY!? It feels like someone is stabbing my insides and you're asking about my stress? Of course, that's causing me stress! I used the term "stabbing"!

If you haven't figured it out at this point, I'm talking about myself. And that doctor's question about stress wasn't actually uncalled for—it was relevant, even if it wasn't exactly put as delicately as it could have been.

But 17-year-old me was convinced I wasn't stressed. *The pain* was causing me stress, sure, but I was fine. Everything was fine. (Reader, everything was not fine.)

Not convinced that I was telling the whole truth, the doctor asked me what was going on in my life at that moment. Well, I was about to head into final exam season. I was waiting to hear back from the colleges I had applied to. I was getting ready to embark on a big, scary, exciting, unknown stage of my life that would most likely take me far away from my family and friends. But, no, everything was cool—not stressed at all.

After several tests to rule out a few other diagnoses, I was told the pain was most likely caused by IBS. And over a decade later spent experiencing many bouts of stomach pain and other digestive woes, often coinciding conveniently with intense periods of stress and anxiety, I'm pretty confident that that was the right call.

I understand why it's a hard pill to swallow that stress could be a contributing or primary factor in our physical symptoms. It certainly was for me. I mean, what if my doctor had been so convinced that my stress was the major factor that they didn't order certain tests? What if I were a patient who had already been routinely dismissed by her doctor? When your concerns have been dismissed before—which happens often and disproportionately to people in marginalized groups—it's a lot harder to accept an answer that ends with "or it might be stress." Sometimes, it's not.

This paradox—that your mind and body are often connected and that sometimes that fact is used to dismiss larger health concerns—is an uncomfortable one, but it's one that I think is important to keep in mind when we're listening to our bodies. It's also something that physicians are hopefully acutely aware of as they interact with patients, too.

"If you are trying to tell someone who has pain that they also have anxiety and you're not quite right, it is going to sound like you told the person it's in their heads," says Gunter.

But two things can be true—especially when it comes to your body. You can have chronic pain *and* anxiety. That's a possibility, but it's far from the only possibility. It's also a possibility that your anxiety contributes to your pain, just as it's a possibility that the two are entirely unrelated or that some other not-yet-diagnosed ailment is actually contributing to both.

When listening to your body, be aware of this paradox. Know that it is possible for your mental health to affect your physical health and vice versa in ways that even researchers don't always fully understand. But also know that if your doctor is not willing to explain to you why that may be the case and what else they are doing to investigate and treat your symptoms, then they are not doing their job. And you are, hopefully, able to find someone else who can.

KNOW THAT SOMETIMES, YOUR BODY JUST STRAIGHT UP FUCKS WITH YOU.

Otherwise known as a panic attack. If you've ever had a panic attack, you know that your body is capable of drumming up some truly awful symptoms, pretty much on demand.

Sweating, shaking, tingling, numbness, dizziness, chills, nausea, heart palpitations, struggling to breathe, and the overwhelming certainty that you are 100% dying—yeah, those can all be symptoms of a panic attack.

The first time I had a panic attack, I thought I was having an allergic reaction, a stroke, or something else that was probably fatal. Unfortunately, one panic attack turned into many, which turned into a lot of really rough times throughout college and at least one embarrassing trip to the ER in the middle of the night.

Actually, scratch that—I take back the embarrassing part. Why do we assume it's embarrassing to seek help for very real, very terrifying physical sensations? My guess is that it's because most people don't know what causes panic attacks, so they see it as someone overreacting or just being dramatic. I'm going to stop short of wishing a panic attack on everyone—but, seriously, if you had one, you would get it—and instead explain what's actually going on in the body when you experience one. Once I started researching and reporting on panic attacks, my own actually became much less frequent and much more manageable.

When our body perceives a threat, we go into what's called fight-or-flight mode, which refers to a series of physiological changes thought to be caused by the release of adrenaline. Your heart starts beating faster, your breathing becomes quicker, your muscles tense up, your blood flow is redirected from your extremities to your big muscle groups. All of this would be super helpful if you actually needed to fight or flee.

"All these things are good—they're *unpleasant*—which is good because that's going to motivate you to escape," explains Abramowitz. "It's like an alarm going off. Alarms *should* be unpleasant."

Fair. But why the hell is this alarm going off when you're just lying in bed or walking down the street? Yep, that's the mystery. Panic attacks are thought to always be triggered by *something,* but that doesn't always mean it's *something obvious.* That something is what kicked off a cascade of very real physiological changes that your mind interprets (rightfully) as an alarm. And once the alarm starts going off, you start (rightfully) panicking.

It's not uncommon during a panic attack to feel an overwhelming sense of dread. I mean some absolute certainty that this is the end for you. It's awful. Try to think of that as your panicked mind's confirmation bias—it's quickly surveying the situation and reporting back: *Yep, you're probably dying.* Again, this is frustratingly, inexplicably typical as far as panic attacks are concerned.

"It's not only the physical stuff, but there's also a change in your mental functioning as well," explains Abramowitz. "We pay attention to the threat, and this is where hypervigilance comes in. If the threat is coming from outside—like a saber-toothed tiger—the person scans the environment. If the threat is coming from within—'Oh no, I'm having a heart attack! Oh no, I have the virus!'—then we're scanning the internal environment. And what a panic attack is is really when a person starts scanning their body, notices their heart's racing, [assumes] 'Oh my god, I'm having a heart attack,' and that cues off the fight-or-flight response. And then their heart gets even faster and they work themselves into this tizzy, when in fact the only thing that's happening is the fight-or-flight response."

Of course, this is all a very long, drawn out explanation of what's happening in the span of—typically—a very short period of time. When you're in one, you don't know that these symptoms are being caused by your reaction to your fight-or-flight response, which was triggered by who knows what. All you know is what you're feeling at that moment. All you know is that these symptoms are real. They are happening. They are not in your head.

Understanding panic attacks isn't a cure for panic attacks—not by any means. But knowing why and how they happen can be really powerful ammunition the next time you're experiencing one. It demystifies them a little. You know your body has some tricks up its sleeve, and it'll still probably fool you a few times, but it won't hurt you. It loses a little bit of its shock value. You know how the sausage is made, so to speak.

When I was in my early twenties, I lived in a house in Queens with a few roommates, one of whom thought it would be hilarious to hide a life-size male mannequin he found on the street in random areas of the house to scare us. The first time I came home late at night and turned on the light to see Mannie Quinn sitting at the kitchen table, I thought I was *for sure* going to be murdered. But my discovery meant that I got to hide him next. I chose my other roommate's desk chair in his bedroom, and I gotta say that hearing that shriek was pretty satisfying. Each subsequent time I stumbled upon Mannie I was a little less startled, until eventually finding him under my bed was more annoying than terrifying.

Honestly, the same thing happened with me and panic attacks. Once I understood more about what was going on in my body during those moments of panic, each one was a little less traumatic. I still have one occasionally—just like I would still be startled if that damn mannequin showed up at my apartment nearly a decade later—but I know I'll get through it. You will too. Sometimes, your body just likes to fuck with you.

LEARN HOW TO PUT YOUR THOUGHTS ON TRIAL.

So how do you know the difference between intuition and anxiety when it comes to something feeling off in your body? I realize that it's not enough to say that sometimes a lot of miserable symptoms are not going to point to something concrete, diagnosable, or treatable. That sucks. We want answers!

Here's the thing . . . there is no super simple secret way to figure that out. I really hope you weren't expecting there to be, because I'd hate to disappoint you. But this also doesn't mean that you can't try to get closer to the truth. To do that, you have to go all Judge Judy on your ass, or . . . your vagina, or whatever body part is stressing you out at the moment.

You have to challenge yourself like Judge Judy confronts a plaintiff who doesn't seem to be telling the whole story. You have to get all the facts, look at all the evidence, cross-examine the witness. (Guys, I have no idea how courts work.) Basically, you have to put your thoughts on trial. According to Abramowitz, this technique is actually part of the approach used in cognitive behavioral therapy (CBT), often considered the gold standard of treatment for anxiety, OCD, and related disorders.

It might seem ridiculous at first. You might be saying, "Um, I know what I know." Fair. And I have no doubt that you have been paying attention to your body and you do know what's going on in there. But this is also true: We are often very unreliable experts. We forget stuff. We misremember shit. We overestimate risk. We're rife with biases. We're quick to connect the dots in ways that don't always make sense but seem convenient, and some of us don't even know our vaginas from our vulvas. We may be the experts of our own bodies, but we are not always reliable narrators of what goes on inside of them. Hence, trial.

Let's say you've been noticing some random spotting and discomfort lately and you're freaking out that it could be something serious, like cervical cancer. Your first urge is to Google "cervical cancer symptoms," cross-reference all of your own symptoms with the information that pops up, look up the prevalence of cervical cancer in people your age, decide that you can definitely be one of the 8 in 100,000 women diagnosed with cervical cancer each year, and continue to go down a rabbit hole of information that tells you about diagnosis, treatment, prognosis, etc.[32] Tell me, are you calmer now? Yeah, didn't think so. Let's rewind and try that again.

So you've been noticing some random spotting and discomfort lately and you're freaking out that it could be something serious, like cervical cancer. Now, if you're someone who tends to get anxious about their body, usually overestimates their risk for serious diseases, and can spend the better part of an evening searching their symptoms, I'm going to suggest you try putting your thoughts on trial before you turn to the internet.

Here's what that line of questioning might look like:

- Why do I think I might have cervical cancer?

- What evidence do I have that makes me think I have cervical cancer?

- What evidence do I have that suggests that I don't have it?

- What alternate explanations could there be?

- Have I thought that I had cancer before? What happened those times?

This type of questioning is also referred to as Socratic questioning, and it's a tool often used in CBT to help people identify and challenge their beliefs and thought processes. It basically helps to shift your perspective and zoom out from your initial assumptions.

What I would *not* recommend is using the internet to help you answer any of these questions. The point is to put your own thoughts and assumptions on trial—not to bolster your confirmation bias with CDC data. Trust me, I know how hard it is to fight that temptation. When I have an assumption in my head, the journalist in me wants to immediately start researching and gathering evidence that either confirms or refutes those beliefs. Try not to do this. Instead, use this line of questioning to view your *concerns* a little more objectively—like if your best friend came to you with the same worry. I happen to be lucky enough to have a best friend who often comes to me with the same kind of tell-me-if-this-sounds-ridiculous health and body questions that I throw at her, so I've had a lot of practice. And it gets easier with practice, trust me.

THE 24-HOUR RULE

Have you ever spent the better part of a night tossing and turning, stressing about something that seemed so huge and scary and undeniable, only to finally tire yourself out and wake up feeling . . . mostly fine? Yeah, me too. Anxiety sure is a tricky bitch like that.

Somewhere along my health anxiety journey, I instituted a 24-hour rule. It's exactly what it sounds like: a 24-hour moratorium on worrying about whatever latest odd body thing I'm currently stressing about—as long as I'm not actually debilitated or bleeding or on fire. If I still feel the same after that break, I'll do something about it. Most times, I don't even remember to check back in on myself 24 hours later.

It's a huge practice of self-restraint, for sure. But, honestly, the planner in me kind of loves that I'm basically scheduling time into my calendar to panic. And if, when the time comes, I don't still feel like panicking, even better! If you decide to try this, you might notice the same thing I did: my record of holy-shit-I'm-dying moments that actually persisted past the 24-hour rule is shockingly low. And that realization motivates me to keep this rule going.

There are a few ways you can do this, so I suggest playing around until you find something that works for you. Maybe you literally set an alarm for 24 hours later. Maybe you write down your concerns on a sheet of paper and then put that paper somewhere you won't look for at least 24 hours. Maybe you just make a mental note. The goal is just to somehow signal to yourself that this is something you are going to put out of your mind for a bit. It's off-limits for now. If there's reason to panic, you'll still be able to do so tomorrow. The key is to make yourself pause, take a breath, and assess the situation when you aren't in as anxious a state as you are right now. It's almost like training yourself to not see every single discomfort as an emergency.

It reminds me of something my friend Melanie told me shortly after the coronavirus pandemic hit the northeastern United States in spring 2020. She was doing her medical residency at a hospital in Pennsylvania and occasionally worked the call center. During this time, when she answered the phones, she always said, "What is your emergency?" At times, people were caught off guard, stumbling a bit before saying, "Well, it's not exactly an emergency I guess, but . . ." It was a subtle way to identify the true medical emergencies while the world was, in general, in a state of emergency. Ever since she told me that story, I've thought about it whenever I'm starting to spiral into worst-case-scenario territory for something I literally just noticed.

What is your emergency?

If I can't answer that without stumbling, I institute the 24-hour rule.

KNOW THAT SOME FLUCTUATION IS JUST PART OF HAVING A BODY.

Here's the thing, there is so much weird shit that happens in your body that turns out to be nothing. That certainly doesn't mean that you should dismiss everything you feel, but it's an important reminder that health isn't defined by the absence of any symptoms at all. Your body's internal processes are occasionally going to be noticeable to you—like gas, muscle soreness, or ovulation. And yes, all of those typical bodily functions can also sometimes—rarely—spell trouble. That's the frustrating paradox that we have to live with. But in the meantime, remember that some bumps and blips within your body are just par for the course.

As Abramowitz explains: "Our bodies are noisy. And they normally do all sorts of little stuff here and there to maintain homeostasis and adjust themselves based on the temperature, what you've eaten, or all sorts of little things. And that doesn't mean that there's a problem. It's just your body just doing its thing to stay alive."

But when we're hypervigilant about our bodies, those little body noises can be so loud they drown out everything else. And, believe it or not, your attention can actually add fuel to the anxiety fire.

"It's kind of like if I said I want you to think about your left pinky toe right now," explains Yip. "Even though you hadn't felt it, all of the sudden, even without moving it, you feel it more loudly because you're paying more attention to it. It's about what you're allowing into your awareness."

When we're hyperaware of something that feels off about our bodies, it often appears to be more salient. And if we start catastrophizing about it, our adrenaline can start flowing, and our fight-or-flight response can kick in, which can lead to even more physiological changes for us to freak out about.

This doesn't mean it's as simple as turning down a dial on your hypervigilance. If we could do that, this book would be a lot shorter. So instead, I want you to just try to remember that bodies can be noisy. And hypervigilance can often interpret that noise as something terrifying, which pushes you into the health-stress spiral. Try to spot hypervigilance just as quickly as you're able to spot those body blips.

For me, I've noticed my hypervigilance tends to be strongest when I'm stressed, overwhelmed, sleep-deprived, or anxious about literally anything.

It's almost as if my fuse is shorter, or I'm just feeling primed for chaos. At those times, the littlest thing can send me spiraling. But noticing this has made it a little bit easier for me to stop before it starts snowballing.

Think for a second about the last time that you freaked out about something going on with your body that actually turned out to be nothing. I'm willing to bet you were going through some shit at the time, too. Maybe you were super stressed. Maybe your anxiety was at a level 17. Maybe you were drinking way more caffeine than usual or sleeping way less. Maybe there was a viral pandemic going on. The next time you're feeling calm after one of those instances, try journaling about what *else* was going on in your life at the time. You might find some interesting patterns of your own that you can use to keep your hypervigilance in check. Hopefully, you can get to a place where you can tell those random body noises to hush so you can get on with your life.

TRY TO GET COMFORTABLE WITH UNCERTAINTY.

What you'll find when you start putting your anxious health thoughts on trial is that often you'll end up with an answer like: It's *probably* nothing. And that is quite possibly the most frustrating answer for someone with anxiety. We absolutely hate uncertainty. We can't deal with it. That's why we so often go searching for answers online—because we're looking for literally any semblance of reassurance.

But learning to get comfortable with some uncertainty is crucial if you deal with health anxiety the way I do. No amount of research or reading is going to completely take the uncertainty away. If my story doesn't reinforce that, I don't know what will.

Learning to live with that uncertainty is another mainstay of CBT for anxiety disorders. So what does it mean to get comfortable with uncertainty around your health?

- It means not seeking reassurance every time we think we have an illness.

- It means not Googling the symptoms of said illness to see how many of them you can check off.

- It means realizing that even when we get some reassurance—from a search engine, a doctor, a test result—we often still aren't satisfied.

- It means accepting that life is filled with uncertainty and that we cannot let the fear of not knowing exactly how this will turn out stop us from moving forward.

"Part of treatment is to be able to entertain uncertainty, to embrace that uncertainty that we never know," says Yip. "And that's part of the interesting part of life, right? Imagine if you go through life knowing exactly what's going to happen every single moment."

While I responded to Yip with "Ha, exactly!" I was really thinking, *Um, actually, that would be great. Is that an option?*

So, yeah, that's where I am. And maybe that's where you are, too. That's alright—learning to live with uncertainty is really freaking hard. I don't want to give the impression that it's easy or something you do once. This isn't just mind over matter—this is going to take work.

If this is something you're struggling with, please remember that there are people whose whole job it is to help. Yip suggests looking for a therapist who specializes in CBT for anxiety disorders. And if you're not sure where to start, don't worry—we'll get to that in chapter 8.

CHAPTER 5

How to decode the latest health headlines

SETTLE IN, FOLKS, BECAUSE THIS CHAPTER IS A LONG ONE, and I'm gonna tell you why.

When I first sat down to write this book, I was really excited about this chapter, because it covers a topic I could talk about all day long. I mean, come on . . . The ways that clickbait headlines and sloppy reporting lead people to believe—and share!—health misinformation? That's 100% my soapbox. Telling people that it's totally possible to write health content that is super compelling and fun while also still being accurate and responsible? That's 100% my jam.

I was ready to crush this chapter. I was ready to hand over my tools and tricks so you could be way more discerning the next time your friend from high school shares an article about tequila helping you lose weight or champagne boosting your memory. I actually remember telling a friend that I could write this chapter in my sleep.

And then the coronavirus pandemic happened—and the stakes got infinitely higher.

When I set out to write this book, most people were already getting the majority of their health information from some form of media—typically online. But the type of health content most people were consuming from the media was a little different. It was still the kind of thing that could influence the way you take care of your body—like an article about bacon causing cancer or one about cranberry juice treating UTIs. But my hunch is that the vast majority of people were interacting with health messaging like this on a pretty casual basis. Were there some people who radically changed their lifestyles as a result of health news they saw on TV or Facebook? Yeah, of course. But my guess is that sort of reaction was pretty limited, and it was mostly happening among a pretty specific demographic of people. You know, the wellness consumer. They have a subscription to *Women's Health* or *Men's Health*. They follow Well+Good on Instagram. They have a jade roller. They take probiotics. You know the people I mean. It's me. It's you. It's anyone you thought of when you saw this book.

Anyway, that's the person I was initially writing it for: the person who already gets a lot of their fitness, nutrition, and self-care intel from wellness media. My goal was to make that process easier, less predatory, more empowering. It already felt like a lofty goal considering the amount of garbage health information that was out there.

And then the coronavirus pandemic happened—and the stakes got infinitely higher.

Suddenly we weren't just relying on the media for occasional health content that we may or may not use in the future. And it wasn't just a small demographic of people engaging with this content. The entire country—and the world—was now relying on the media for crucial updates on where and how this virus was spreading, not to mention necessary information on how to tweak basically every aspect of our lives in order to stay safe. Of course, click-bait headlines and sloppy reporting persisted—and don't even get me started on the memes. Before this, I thought misleading headlines about "super gonorrhea" were among the most irresponsible examples of health journalism.

But now? I'm going to need a bigger soapbox.

I'm still going to give you actionable ways to be more discerning, more skeptical, and more empowered when it comes to the types of health messages you see every day. And I'm still going to call out misleading reporting on nutrition or sexual health as incredibly irresponsible, because it is. But I realize things have changed now. And I trust you do, too.

So I hope you'll keep that in mind and use these tips not just to make sense of the headlines about celery juice or CBD oils—ah, what a simpler time—but also on the bigger public health news that you maybe never had to interact with before. As we've all seen, what's trending in the health news space will continue to change in very unpredictable ways. Take it from me: whatever the headlines say is killing you or curing you when you sign your book deal may be vastly different from what's killing you or curing you when you sit down to write it.

With all that in mind, the following sections are meant to guide you in better deciphering and digesting whatever pops up in the health headlines next—because who knows what will be trending by the time this book ends up in your hands. No matter what it is—and, man, I hope it's not murder hornets; I feel like those are going to make a comeback—I hope the advice here will give you the critical thinking skills needed to react to it in a way that's confident, capable, and calm. (Unless it's actually murder hornets—then you have my permission to panic.)

Consider the source.

If you take just one thing away from this chapter—or, honestly, this whole book—let it be this: when it comes to health information, always consider the source. I firmly believe that the biggest advantage that I have over the average wellness con-

> *When it comes to health information, always consider the source.*

sumer isn't my ability to parse through jargon-y journal articles or complicated data—it's my experience tracking down the right sources. It's being able to make an informed judgment about when a source is reputable and trustworthy . . . or not.

> **What I want you to remember is that reach does not equal expertise.**

This is so important because the reality is that anyone with access to the internet can create and share health information. Seriously, anyone! Think about the most heinous, ill-informed, ignorant person you can imagine. Yeah, even them. They can come up with some bullshit tincture, say that they've successfully treated tons of people with it, and create a campaign for this "miracle cure." They might reach three people, or, with enough luck and connections, they might reach millions. Now, if you knew this person were full of shit, that would be really hard to watch, right? But when you don't have any previous knowledge of that person and what they're selling, it can be a lot harder to spot the bullshit. Let me help with that.

What I want you to remember is that reach does not equal expertise. Too often we see someone giving an interview on TV or posting something on social media, and we think, *Well, they must be legit; otherwise the show wouldn't book them.* Or *They must know what they're talking about; otherwise 1.3 million people wouldn't have shared this.* Man, I really wish those assumptions were true. Unfortunately, they just aren't.

There's one simple reason that people get booked on TV shows and start trending on social media even if they have absolutely no expertise or authority on the topic at hand: it's because their message is engaging. If someone has something to say that is surprising or exciting or polarizing or affirming or otherwise likely to rile people up, that message is probably going to go places. TV pundits will want to elevate it, because it will make their audiences tune in. Ordinary people will want to share it, retweet it, link-in-bio-it so that their followers know where they stand. We see this happen every single day.

Things don't go viral because they're accurate or they're coming from a reliable source. They go viral because people identify with the message or the messenger on a visceral level—one that compels them to say "Yes, this!" and hit share before they even take a closer look at what they're sharing.

Reach does not equal expertise. So how else can you tell if a source is trustworthy, if they're a legitimate, authoritative supplier of this information? Well, it depends on the kind of source that you're dealing with. Below are some checklists that can help you identify a legitimate source of health information, depending on where you're getting it:

IF IT'S A PERSON

What are their qualifications to give information and advice on this topic? What you're looking for here are things like:

- **DEGREES FROM ACCREDITED INSTITUTIONS:** Someone with an MPH (Master of Public Health) from the Yale School of Public Health is probably a fantastic source *on public health.* But if they're giving advice about diagnosing and treating something like asthma or allergies or athlete's foot, you're probably going to want that person to have a medical degree like an MD or a DO.

- **BOARD CERTIFICATION:** If someone is board certified in a specialty—like dermatology or gynecology—that means they've gone through additional extensive training in that particular area. Personally, I want to get my vagina advice from someone who is board certified in obstetrics and gynecology, but that's just me. (Hot tip: You can check if your doctor is board certified by going to certificationmatters.org.)

- **AFFILIATIONS OR CERTIFICATIONS WITH REPUTABLE ORGANIZATIONS IN THIS FIELD:** If the expert isn't a medical doctor, you can check to see if they're affiliated or certified through other important organizations in their industry. For instance, certification with the American Association of Sexuality Educators, Counselors and Therapists (AASECT) is considered the gold standard for sex therapists.

O **DOCUMENTED EXPERIENCE WITH THIS TOPIC:** If they're speaking about treatment options, do they actually treat patients with this condition, or are they in an adjacent field that doesn't have the hands-on experience that would be helpful here?

O **PREVIOUS ACCLAIM AS AN EXPERT ON THIS TOPIC:** This isn't necessary, especially if someone is just starting out in their career, but it's a pretty good sign if someone has already written books or led speaking engagements around this subject. That said, I would be wary of this *without* the other qualifications on this list. Like I said, it's possible for someone to become an "expert" on something in the public eye without actually having the required experience to back it up.

O **NO SHADY MOTIVES THAT YOU CAN SEE:** Now this one is tricky, because if you have a conspiratorial worldview, it's possible you can find a shady motive in everyone. But what I generally mean by this is: do they seem disproportionately focused on trying to promote something other than general good health practices? For example, I've spoken to many experts over the years that met all of the previous qualifications, but they were also selling products or services that just didn't pass the gut check (more on that in chapter 6). Or sometimes they also happened to be a spokesperson for a certain pharmaceutical company, and the persistence with which they snuck mentions of these products or drugs into our conversations was a little unsettling to the journalist in me. Again, if they meet all the other criteria on this list, I wouldn't necessarily discount them, but I probably wouldn't use them as a source about treatments, for instance, if they were a known spokesperson for one specific brand. If you suspect a conflict of interest, do some digging, ask questions, and trust your gut.

IF IT'S A MEDIA OUTLET

This all comes down to asking yourself why you should trust them to report accurately and responsibly on this topic. Here are some things you should consider:

- **THE OUTLET'S REPUTATION:** Is this a well-known brand owned by a big, legacy media company, or is it a small blog that's been around for a year? One isn't always more trustworthy than the other, but an established brand is likely to have more guidelines and standards in place than a personal blog.

- **THE WRITER:** Is there a byline on the article? Can you find out more about the writer, like if they cover this topic regularly or have specialized training in this subject? If there's no byline, do you feel comfortable taking this kind of information from an unknown source?

- **THE BRAND'S TRACK RECORD IN COVERING THIS TOPIC:** Health and science reporting is very different than, say, the crime beat or foreign affairs. Those all require, ideally, subject matter experts who are trained and experienced in that type of reporting. So when looking for health information, I would suggest looking to the outlets and authors that have a history of covering this responsibly.

- **THEIR SOURCING:** Do they use reputable sources? (I'll cover exactly what that looks like in a bit.) And do they show their work? Can you plainly see where they're getting their information so that you can verify it yourself? If I can't easily confirm the facts and claims in an article because they aren't making it clear where their information comes from, I don't trust it.

○ **ANY POTENTIAL CONFLICTS OF INTEREST:** This one is tricky because it can be really hard to gauge what these are and if they even impact the content you're reading. For instance, you might see that a health website has ads for a pharmaceutical company and assume that they can't be objective, trustworthy reporters. I can totally understand that assumption, but I can also tell you that the degree to which advertisers exert influence over the content that media brands put out can vary *widely*—both from publication to publication and from article to article.

Unfortunately, there's not a lot of transparency on this, but I can say from experience that, most times, the ads that run along the side of an article are handled by a department fully separate from the writers writing the articles. The most common ad-edit conflict I have witnessed was one where the advertiser *didn't* want to be around certain articles—like an article that talks about the side effects of their drug or one that talks about sex. In that case, someone outside of the editorial team would just remove that ad from the article in question. The writer was often never even told. But that doesn't mean that larger conflicts of interest or shady advertiser interference never happen at media companies. They certainly do.

My advice would be to pay attention to the advertising that you see on the site as a whole, especially if you see the same one over and over again. This could show you the types of companies they align with. (Are their ads mostly for FDA-approved medications or herbal detox teas? Do they have ads for a certain political party?) Or it might actually signal that you're looking at a sponsored "hub" of content created specifically at an advertiser's request. You can also look into where their funding comes from. (Are they backed by a privately held publishing company or a political or religious organization? Are they a nonprofit? Are they affiliated with a hospital?)

IF IT'S A MEME

Nope. Stop. Please do not trust any health information in meme form unless it was actually created by a reputable person or media outlet. In that case, see above to determine if they're a trustworthy source. And even then, remember that most health information is a little too complicated to be captured in full in a meme. Trust me, I've tried.

Then, check your source's sources.

I'm not saying that you can only ever get your health information straight from thoroughly vetted doctors and award-winning science publications. I realize that's not how most of us find our workouts, our nutritious recipes, or our healthy life hacks.

I get it—I was a health journalist at BuzzFeed at a time when most people still considered it a website consisting solely of cats and listicles. And I had so many health articles at BuzzFeed go viral. I was giddy every time one of my posts earned the coveted viral badge—a literal badge of honor that popped up on the top of the article when it was trending. Some of my articles racked up millions of views in just days. Every day I couldn't believe that I was reaching that huge of an audience. But remember, reach does not equal expertise.

Now, I like to think that I was a pretty fantastic health journalist, even though my articles ranged from reporting on epidemiological research to a little bit lighter topics, like "24 Dog Pictures That Will Make You Say 'Me on My Period'" and "21 Sex Tips That Aren't Bullshit" (both of which also got the viral badge, thankyouverymuch). When I was taking on a more serious topic—like sexually transmitted infections, birth control efficacy, health disparities, or reproductive rights—I did not take this responsibility lightly. I was fully aware that there were more appropriate places for people to get their health information than BuzzFeed—like the CDC, the NIH, the Guttmacher Institute, and Planned Parenthood, just to name a few. But I also knew that most people weren't doing that. They didn't know where to turn or what to trust. But for some reason, they turned to and trusted BuzzFeed. So I made it my job to introduce readers to those more appropriate sources through my reporting.

I became friendly with a press officer over at the CDC and reached out to them often. And whenever I wrote about CDC data, I made sure to connect with one of their researchers to chat through it so I didn't accidentally misinterpret a table, misattribute a stat, or make any broad generalizations that weren't supported by their findings. I did the same thing when using data from other major medical organizations. I may not have been writing for a medical institution, but I was doing my best to work *with* them to get important health information out there. At one point, I remember telling a colleague that the thing I appreciated most about my job was getting to surprise this massive, cat-loving audience with genuinely helpful health information that they may not have otherwise gotten.

> *What I'm saying is that it's absolutely possible for you to get your health news and information from the outlets that you already know and trust and are comfortable with—as long as you're paying attention to the way they source their information.*

What I'm saying is that it's absolutely possible for you to get your health news and information from the outlets that you already know and trust and are comfortable with—as long as you're paying attention to the way they source their information.

Unfortunately, not everyone knows to do this. I often have to fact-check my own mother on Facebook anytime she shares a meme with a statistic or claim that is just egregiously false.

"Well, I thought it was true!" she says.

Honestly, fair. We should be able to trust the information we're receiving, but the unfortunate reality is that the onus is often on the reader to investigate whether or not the information they're getting is accurate. And that's especially the case with health information.

So how can you do this in the least time-consuming way possible? I have a very simple tip, and it involves a concept you learned way back in elementary school. *Look for the primary sources.* If you can't find the primary source—let alone verify it—I'd highly suggest getting your health information elsewhere.

You probably learned about primary and secondary sources a very long time ago, so don't be embarrassed if you need a quick refresher.

- **PRIMARY SOURCES** are as close to the original information as possible. The most common examples would be firsthand accounts of something or original works—like a speech, a memoir, or a government document.

- **SECONDARY SOURCES** are reporting or commenting on a primary source. Common examples would be a newspaper article on a politician's speech or a documentary about someone's life.

Let me give a more relatable example. A primary source would be a celebrity's Instagram post showing off a freckle that turned out to be cancer, coupled with her caption explaining her diagnosis. It's her firsthand account of what happened. But when BuzzFeed writes a story about that celebrity's cancer diagnosis, that article is a secondary source—even if they embed the Instagram post into the article so you can see it.

That may sound like a silly example, but it's actually a pretty great illustration of celebrity health reporting done right . . . and no, I'm not just saying that because I was the BuzzFeed health editor back in the day. It's because the reporter is very clearly directing readers to the primary source. The reader can quickly access the original information. They can go read the caption and see for themselves if this celebrity actually does say she has cancer or not. In essence, the reporter is showing you the receipts. So as long as the writer is also reporting on the Instagram post accurately and responsibly and not throwing in a bunch of bogus speculation about what caused the cancer or what treatments she might seek, then this article gets an *A* from me. Good job, hypothetical reporter! See, checking if the health news you're consuming is legit or not can be as simple as that.

But it can also get a little more complicated. Sometimes the primary source is harder to find than we expect. This doesn't mean the article or video is bogus, but it's usually not a great sign.

Here's a hypothetical example that could very well actually exist somewhere on the internet: You're watching a video comparing the COVID-19 pandemic to the seasonal flu. Maybe it's on a major news channel and contains an interview with a doctor who treats the flu, so it all seems pretty legit. The doctor says that the flu kills over 60,000 people in the United States in just one year. This all sounds pretty trustworthy, right? You've got a major network that covers health often. You've got a doctor who's seen some shit. He's gotta be a primary source, right? Can't you just accept this as fact, share it with your friends, and move on with your life?

I know I'm not going to make friends with this but . . . No. I'm sorry. You can't. Here's what you would find if you took that video and went hunting for a primary source . . .

First, you should know that doctors and researchers aren't always primary sources—even though we typically assume they are. I know, they're the experts. But experts can be both primary and secondary sources. If a doctor is talking about treating their own patients or about research they themselves conducted, they would be a primary source. But if they're telling you that over 60,000 people die from the flu in one year, they would be the secondary source—unless they were literally the person who tallied up over 60,000 deaths, and I'm guessing they're not. The real primary source of that information would be the mortality data from the CDC. If you didn't know that off the top of your head, that's fine. You can simply Google "how many people die from the flu in the United States" and the CDC should be up near the top of your search results.

Now that we've found the primary source, it's time for a quick verification: Does this source confirm what you read, saw, or heard in the media? In this case, the answer is both yes and no. If you followed that trail and clicked on that link for the CDC, you'd find a page titled: "Disease Burden of Influenza."[33] (Sexy, right? CDC, y'all need better copywriters. Call me.) On that page, you'd find a table documenting how bad the last several flu seasons have been. The table lists the number of illnesses, the number of medical visits, the number of hospitalizations, and the number of deaths for each flu season between 2010 and 2019. Let's see if we can find anything that confirms that over 60,000 people die per year from the flu.

Ah, okay, here we go: In the 2017–2018 flu season, there were an estimated 61,000 deaths. But wait! There's an asterisk!

That asterisk says that estimates from the 2017–2018 flu season "are preliminary and may change as data are finalized." Okay, well the doctor on the video didn't mention that. You'll also notice on that page that there's a link to a whole other page titled "How CDC Estimates the Burden of Seasonal Influenza in the U.S."[34] Yep, a whole page. And it's long. The gist is that the number of flu deaths that are thrown around are actually estimates based on mathematical models that take into consideration a lot of different factors, like the amount of people who die from flu-related complications like pneumonia or stroke who have those conditions listed on their death certificates rather than influenza. So even this primary source isn't super precise, but it's what we've got.

But here's the clincher: On that table listing the estimated flu deaths from each flu season, you'll notice that the 2017–2018 flu season was an outlier. The estimated flu deaths per year actually ranged from 12,000 in the 2011–2012 flu season to 61,000 in the 2017–2018 flu season. Here's a closer look:

FLU SEASON	Estimated Deaths Attributed to Seasonal Influenza
2010–2011	37,000
2011–2012	12,000
2012–2013	43,000
2013–2014	38,000
2014–2015	51,000
2015–2016	23,000
2016–2017	38,000
2017–2018	61,000
2018–2019	34,000

Source: Disease Burden of Influenza, CDC

Yeah, the doctor in the video didn't mention that either.

This is what you get when a vague secondary source leaves you to go fishing for primary sources. In most cases, you're getting a half-baked story, lacking all those little nuances you would hope to get from legitimate health reporting. Think of it like playing a game of telephone. The more steps you have to take between what you're consuming and what actually happened, the more opportunities a message has to get lost in translation. Technically the doctor in the video wasn't lying—they just weren't telling the whole story. Without digging around for the rest of the context, you might have believed that every single year, more than 60,000 people in the U.S. die from the flu. And that's just not true.

This is where highly trained health journalists—and their editors—come in. They're the people who won't let a story run without checking out that stat the doctor mentioned because they know that the doctor isn't the primary source. Remember, that's the journalist's job. It's not your job to have to do all that fact-checking every time you're exposed to health messages. I totally understand that you don't want to work that hard: you're not getting paid for it.

So do you really need to play Veronica Mars every time you read a health article? Hell no. Who has the time? But if this is information that you're planning on applying to your life in some meaningful way or if this is information you want to share with your own circle, then yes, I do expect you to verify it yourself.

I promise it gets easier and quicker with time. When a version of this example happened to me recently, it took me about five minutes to fact-check the Facebook post in question. It's something you'll get more comfortable with the more you do it. And isn't it worth it to know where your health information is coming from? Isn't it worth it to know you aren't spreading lies to your friends and family?

Never trust the phrase "Research shows . . ."

If there's one phrase that should stop you in your tracks when you're reading a health article, it's "Research shows . . ." I know what you're thinking: *Lady, you just said research was a good thing and that we should trust it over people just saying whatever they want.* True. But again, you need to see the receipts. And way too often, writers don't leave you the receipts. Sometimes, they don't even read the receipts.

Here's what I mean: Health writers often like to drop in a "research shows" to add credibility to their reporting. Suddenly an article about why you should masturbate more is legit science journalism because they found a study to back up their claims. Except . . . does that study actually back up those claims? A lot of times, it doesn't.

Let's say the writer wants to find some research that reinforces what they're saying in their piece, so they run some searches on things like "study on masturbation and happiness." Google does its thing and maybe serves up something similar, like a study on happiness and sex. The writer skims the study abstract. (That's the introduction paragraph that very, very briefly summarizes the findings. And it's typically free, whereas the full text of the study is usually behind a paywall.) Or maybe they just read an article or press release about this research, rather than reading the research itself. The writer decides that the study basically backs up what they're trying to say, and they plug it into the story with a line like: "Research shows rubbing one out can actually boost your mood!" But what if that study was actually looking at the sex habits and happiness scores of 20 college-aged men, and your article is about why women should masturbate more? The research did not show that.

As a busy editor, I used to keep tabs on this by asking writers to send me the full-text versions of any studies they referenced in their articles. Sometimes when I was really busy, I even asked them to highlight where exactly in that 42-page PDF I could confirm the claim they were making in their article. If they had a line in their article saying "and research shows masturbation can make us happier," I wanted them to point out exactly what research shows that—and where.

Here's what happened. A lot of writers humored me. They sent me the PDFs they got from the study authors. They highlighted the sections that were relevant. They—by my estimation—actually read the research. But there were also a lot of writers who did not do this. There were writers who, when I asked for the research, said they couldn't track down a copy. Interesting! Tell me how you're gonna say "research says" when you haven't seen that research?

All of this goes to show that you should demand from your health reporters the same thing I demanded from mine: receipts. When someone says, "Research shows . . .," they better *show you the research*. Basically, you want the writer to explain their sources a little bit. A better bet than "Research shows masturbation makes you happier" would be something like: "Research published in the *Journal of Hypothetical Studies* in 2016 looked at 610 women between the ages of 18 and 34 who answered an online survey about their masturbation habits and how happy they felt on a daily basis. Of those survey participants, people who reported masturbating at least once a week also reported being happier, on average, than people who reported masturbating less frequently than that."

You're not always going to get that level of detail, unfortunately. Especially not in print publications or social videos where space is limited and every word counts. So in that case, just keep in mind that when you hear the phrase "research shows" there's a lot more to the story.

Beware of the single study write-up.

This is something that I guarantee you see all the time. I know this because it's something that makes me roll my eyes all the time. You'll see it in your social media feeds, on the 6 o'clock news, on the push alert from your go-to news site. It's a headline that seems important, definitive—groundbreaking even. It looks like some of these very real headlines:

○ **Up to 25 Cups of Coffee a Day Safe for Heart Health, Study Finds**[35]

○ **Cabbage Could Help Fight COVID-19, Study Finds**[36]

○ **Drinking Champagne Is Good for Your Brain and Prevents Memory Loss**[37]

I like to call these Big If True! Headlines. I'm sure you can figure out why.

Sometimes you click on these and read more about it. Other times you don't bother—the headline was enough. But even if you barely give headlines like these a second glance, I'm willing to bet that these messages actually seep into your everyday life and decision-making much more than you think.

Imagine this hypothetical but relatable scenario: You're having drinks with your friends and a topic related to one of those buzzy headlines comes up.

"I think I drink too much coffee," says one friend. "I feel useless without it, but I get jittery when I have too much. Also I'm having trouble sleeping. I probably need to cut down on caffeine, right?"

> *There are very few times that medical experts and researchers would advise the general public to make sweeping changes to their lifestyles based on one single study.*

"*Actually* I just heard that up to 25 cups of coffee a day is totally healthy. There was a whole study on it. So it's probably fine," says another friend, who definitely didn't click on or read the actual article she's referring to—but she saw the headline.

Now, I could walk through each of those headlines and cover all of the nuances of each study or survey in depth to show you the difference between headline and reality, but suffice it to say that the framing in each of those examples is incredibly misleading—for multiple reasons. But the most basic crime is this: the media is hitting you with a bold claim that sounds definitive and science-backed, when in reality it is based on a single study with tons of limitations—because all research has limitations.

There are very few times that medical experts and researchers would advise the general public to make sweeping changes to their lifestyles based on one single study. And yet here we are giving it loads of attention in the media. Why are we like this?

Um, are "laziness and capitalism" too simplistic an answer? Okay, but seriously, in my experience, single-study write-ups are the low-hanging fruit of health and science writing. They're easy and cheap. And from my vantage point in digital media, they often resulted in a lot of traffic. My guess is that television stations and print publications rely on them in a similar fashion: they're quick hits.

When I was a young and inexperienced writer, I wrote a ton of these to meet whatever quota I needed to hit at the time. I was taught to scroll through the health and science press releases every day to see if there was anything that might be interesting for whatever outlet I was writing for. A new psychology study? Perfect. A new survey on sexual preferences? Oh hell yeah. An incredibly preliminary study on a new birth control method that will probably never make it to market? Yes, dibs. Basically, if I could write a grabby-as-hell headline around it, it could run. And it would probably do well.

At the time, I felt like a real health journalist—emailing the study author out in Australia to get a copy of the full study, reading it top to bottom, highlighting it, staying after hours to call up that study author to get a few quotes, and filing it to my editor with a couple of different headline options.

Now, I cringe when I think about how I was essentially writing press releases dressed up as health articles. Even if I included all of the necessary caveats and limitations ("It's worth noting that this study was only done in mice . . ." or "Keep in mind that this survey was funded by Big Cranberry Juice . . ." or "Granted, the survey participants were 60 cisgender, heterosexual, white women at an Ivy League college, so the results may not be generalizable to the broad population . . ."), who knows if the readers took those things to heart. Honestly, who knows if the readers even read the damn article. I was writing headlines that amplified an idea that I knew required 800 words of thorough explanation and yet most people were just going to remember the headline.

My approach to these articles changed throughout my career. As I gained both perspective and decision-making power, I began only covering or assigning stories on one-off studies in the spirit of addressing or debunking a prevailing narrative that was already out there. For instance, something like: "What You Need to Know about All Those Headlines Claiming Champagne Improves Your Memory" or "Does Champagne Actually Improve Your Memory?"

But even then, I realized that tons of people were still just reading the headlines or briefly skimming the articles. And most of us hear only what we want to hear, read only what we want to read. If we want to believe that champagne is a magic brain elixir, that's probably what we're going to take away from the article, even if it's filled with phrasing that assures the reader that that's not what's going on.

I'm not saying that every health and science study you see in the news is actually hot trash. I'm not quite that cynical. But I do want your bullshit alarm to start sounding when you see a Big If True! Headline. I want you to keep in mind that this is probably based on a single study, the results are most likely not applicable to you, and you shouldn't make any life changes based on this information right away.

Spoiler alert, that champagne study was done in "aged rodents."[38] You are not an aged rodent.

Remember that correlation does not equal causation.

This is a lesson that will serve you very well in decoding all sorts of health headlines. It's something I find myself dropping in my family's group chat often, especially when they want my take on some new "miracle" cure or "groundbreaking" study.

For reference, I wrote much of this book at the beginning of the COVID-19 pandemic, when new articles about possible treatments and cures were popping up every single day. This was both exhilarating and exhausting. It was promising to see the best minds in medicine moving so quickly to try to draw any possible conclusions that we could work with to keep people alive. It was also terrifying to see people wholeheartedly believe—and act on—research that was very preliminary and as yet unproven.

Correlation vs. causation was a common theme that kept coming up. I felt like a broken record when saying it to my family and friends. So let's talk about the difference between correlation and causation and why knowing that difference will help you call bullshit on a whole lot of health messaging that you're exposed to every day.

Correlation refers to an observed relationship between two things. It's a pattern, an association, a link. For instance, you might notice a correlation between getting your period and eating massive amounts of chocolate. Or you might notice a correlation between people who like pumpkin spice lattes and people who have Live, Laugh, Love decorations in their house. Or maybe you can't ignore the correlation between drinking coffee and an urgent need to poop. You get the idea. The key is realizing that a correlation just means that these two things seem to be related in some way. You don't know if *A* is causing *B*, if *B* is causing *A*, or if there's actually a *C* that you haven't even noticed that is causing both *A* and *B*.

Causation, on the other hand, refers to a cause-and-effect relationship. This is when you can actually prove that *A* causes *B*. To prove causation, you need a randomized controlled trial, which is where researchers arbitrarily assign an experimental group to one set of conditions and a control group to another set of conditions to try to control for as many biases as possible. The goal is to be as sure as you can be that *A* is truly causing *B*. The thing is, it's not always ethical or possible to carry out this type of study.

Here's why it's so important to know all of this. We're fed correlations all the time in health headlines, and they're often disguised as causations. You'll see a headline touting "One of Your Favorite Foods Causes Cancer" and think, *Well shit.* But does it actually? Most of the time those stories are about observational data showing a link between people who reported eating that food and people who were diagnosed with cancer.

A lot of times this happens because reporters want to get rid of passive voice in their writing. It's something we're taught in journalism school: Don't say "the bill was passed by the senate" when you could say "the senate passed the bill." But when you do this while talking about study findings, you can end up implying causation when there wasn't any. For instance, the headline "Eating cupcakes was associated with a higher risk of cancer" makes every writer want to change it to: "Eating cupcakes caused cancer." The problem is that "was associated with" and "caused" aren't actually interchangeable. The former is clear that this is merely an observed association, whereas the latter implies an established cause-and-effect relationship. Words matter.

> *Correlations aren't always something to dismiss, but I want you to get in the habit of spotting the difference between correlation and causation.*

Correlations aren't always something to dismiss, but I want you to get in the habit of spotting the difference between correlation and causation. If a story is relying on a correlation, recognize the limits of that. Ask questions. A good place to start would be: what are you basing this off of?

For instance, sometimes correlations come from a large body of high-quality, observational research—like everything we know about how smoking cigarettes leads to cancer. As I mentioned, it's not always ethical or possible to carry out randomized controlled trials to prove a cause-and-effect relationship—like knowingly having a group of participants smoke lots of cigarettes to see if they get cancer—but there are other things that researchers look for that would further their case that A is most likely causing B—like nailing down a mechanism of action. This means that they can understand, based on existing research, *how A* could hypothetically *cause B*. Having that mechanism of action to point to can really strengthen some observational research.

But a correlation could also just come from anecdotal evidence, which is considered some of the lowest-quality evidence. Anecdotal evidence relies on personal testimony, and there are a lot of things that can go wrong with that: people can misremember, they can exaggerate, they can let their own biases influence them. So if a correlation is based solely on anecdotal data, I would want to find out things like: How many people reported this? What steps were taken to ensure that people are telling the truth and remembering things accurately? Are there any other possibilities that might be responsible for the association?

Here's another example. My friend and I have a running joke/theory that a certain type of cereal really makes us gassy and bloated. Like, guaranteed. We had no idea why, but we both noticed that whenever we ate it, our stomachs felt like balloons ready to pop. Now, that's a correlation—and a pretty weak one at that since it was only based on two anecdotal reports. But then we mentioned this to a few of our other friends, and they said they noticed the same thing. More anecdotal evidence ensued. But remember, anecdotal data alone is highly suspect. We could all be falling victim to confirmation bias, which means we're only remembering the times that we ate the cereal and were gassy and not all the times that we ate the cereal and weren't gassy, or when we were gassy and didn't eat the cereal. If we could point to a mechanism of action that explains why this cereal makes our stomachs so gassy and swollen, that might help.

Reader, we did. After doing some research—probably when I was procrastinating on a much more important task—I found out that this cereal has a lot of fiber in it. Like, a lot. The U.S. Dietary Guidelines suggest getting 14 grams of fiber for every 1,000 calories in your diet (so, if you're eating around 2,000 calories per day, that would be around 28 grams of fiber), which is way more than most people are actually eating.[39] That is, unless you eat this cereal, which packs almost half the daily recommended amount of fiber for grown adults in one serving—and I don't know anyone who eats *only* the recommended serving size of cereal. And it turns out that consuming too much fiber in one sitting—especially if you aren't drinking enough water with it—is a very well-established way to make you gassy and bloated.[40]

Knowing that my friend and I were 22-year-olds generally eating and drinking like trash when we made this revelation, it makes perfect sense that front-loading our stomachs with fiber every morning was leading to mayhem in our guts.

But without carrying out a randomized controlled trial on this subject—could you imagine the Craigslist ad for that?—it's still technically just a correlation. It's good information to know. And yes, I did change my behavior because of it. (To this day I politely decline that type of cereal.) But I still know it would be irresponsible to publish a headline that says: "Popular Cereal Causes Hella Gas" even though I know people would click on that.

Know the difference between absolute and relative risk.

A lot of headlines talk about risk—like that a certain behavior increases your risk of dying, that one birth control method poses a higher risk of blood clots than another, or that people with purple hair have a lower risk of being boring. You get it.

When you read or hear a story like this, your first question is probably: "Okay, hold up, by how much?" And that's not a bad question. After all, raising your risk of cancer by 2 percent is very different than raising your risk by 200 percent. But, in my opinion, that's not actually the most important question you should be asking. What you should really be asking is: what is the absolute risk?

Let's use an example from a scary headline you've probably seen before: "Birth Control Increases Risk for Deadly Blood Clots."

Terrifying, right? You've no doubt seen several iterations of that headline over the years. It's a topic that gets covered a lot and with good reason because it's something that people should know about. But it's also a headline that fills me with a little bit of rage. I'm willing to bet that even though you've heard this countless times, you probably can't tell me what someone's *actual risk* of developing a blood clot is—on or off birth control.

My rage comes from the media's frequent coverage of relative risk over absolute risk. Often these stories say something to the effect of: "People on the pill are 3x more likely to get a blood clot than people who aren't on it" or "Newer forms of birth control are 1.8x more likely to cause a blood clot than older types." Well, okay, three times more than what? And 1.8 times more than what?! All this tells us is the relative risk, not the absolute risk.

Relative risk lets you know how something affects your risk *compared to* some other alternative. For instance, you might have a 30 percent higher risk of getting hit in the face by a pigeon in New York City than in Atlanta (yes this happened to me, no I don't want to talk about it). As you can see, that only tells you half the story. Your next logical question would be: Well, what's my ACTUAL risk of getting hit in the face with a pigeon in either city? That would be your absolute risk.

In medicine, absolute risk often refers to your risk of developing a disease at some point in your life. So let's say your absolute risk of getting a particular disease is 2 in 100. But let's say you have a genetic predisposition that makes you 50 percent more likely to get that disease. That sure sounds like you are highly likely to get that disease, right? But 50 percent is your relative risk. In this case, a 50 percent increased risk would give you an absolute risk of 3 in 100.

Let's go back to the example of birth control raising your risk of blood clots. According to a 2016 clinical practice guideline from the American Society of Reproductive Medicine (ASRM), the incidence of venous thromboembolism (VTE, the medical term for a blood clot that starts in a vein) is estimated to be between 1 and 5 per 10,000 women per year, outside of pregnancy.[41] That's a 0.01 to 0.05 percent chance of getting a blood clot each year. The risk of VTE is higher in women who are pregnant (5–20 per 10,000 women per year), and it's much higher in women who just gave birth (40–65 per 10,000 women per year).

And yes, the ASRM also noted that plenty of research suggests that birth control can raise your risk of VTE, but that increased risk is still thought to be lower than your risk of VTE while pregnant or postpartum. So the headlines you saw about birth control raising your risk of a blood clot are true—they just don't really help you contextualize your risk in a meaningful way, because they often leave out those absolute risk numbers.

For instance, a 2015 study published in the *BMJ*[42] that was cited in headlines like "Why Are Women Dying From Taking The Pill?"[43] estimated that an additional 6 cases per 10,000 women per year occur as a result of taking birth control with levonorgestrel (an older type of progestin), while an extra 14 cases per 10,000 women per year occur as a result of taking birth control with desogestrel (a newer type of progestin). If you're assuming that your absolute risk is 5 in 10,000 (or 0.05 percent), then an extra 14 cases would raise your absolute risk to 0.19 percent.

But that article only reported on the relative risk—not the absolute risk.

I am not saying that this increased risk is anything to scoff at. Blood clots can be deadly, and if you are one of those 19 in 10,000 women each year that gets one while on the pill, you certainly wouldn't feel like a statistic. All I'm saying is that we deserve to get the full picture when we're fed facts and stats. The media has obviously done a great job of driving home the message that birth control raises the risk of blood clots. But wouldn't it be even better if they drove the full message home?

WHAT DOES *SIGNIFICANT* MEAN, ANYWAY?

You know when you see a story that touts something "significant"—like a drug that significantly reduces the risk of heart failure or a food that is significantly associated with death? That word—*significant*—often gives the whole thing an air of legitimacy. Ah, yes, the findings were significant; guess I'll pay attention to this one!

Let's talk about this for a second, because it may not mean what you think it means. When a piece of research says that a finding was "significant," it just means that the researchers can be sure within a specific level of confidence that their finding was not due to chance. Basically, they can say that they are reasonably certain that whatever their finding was—let's say that their drug lowers the risk of heart failure by 50 percent—this was really a result of the drug and not a random occurrence or due to some other factor they weren't specifically studying. That's what researchers mean by statistical significance.[44]

Clinical significance, on the other hand, refers to how clinically relevant this finding is for doctors and patients. Let's say a study found that a drug lowers the risk of heart failure in rats by 2 percent and the results of that study are statistically significant. Cool, but it's not necessarily *clinically* significant because you are not a rat and you're hoping for a little more than 2 percent improvement if you're going to take a new medication.

So the next time you see the word *significant* in a health story, make sure you know what it's really referring to.

Consider biases, motives, and conflicts of interest.

I am not going to sit here and tell you that the only news you can trust is news that is completely objective and totally unbiased. I genuinely believe that all journalists in all media have some level of inherent bias or motivation that impacts the news stories that they touch—whether it's overt or subtle. We're all human.

But when you think about bias in media, I want you to remember that it's not just in the obvious political leaning of certain media outlets or reporters. It's also in the questions a writer asks their experts and even in the experts that they chose to interview. It's in the way a magazine article is structured or the way a headline is written. It's in the stories that are published—and the ones that aren't. It's in the social media algorithm that shows you only the stories that will rile you up and confirm your deep-seated beliefs.

Some might shake their heads at that, wishing for the "good old days" when "news was just the news." Well, to be fair, I wasn't around for whatever "good old days" these folks are referring to, but my hunch is this: the news wasn't necessarily more objective in the past; there was just less competition for our attention and less transparency in how the media gets made.

And that isn't to say that you shouldn't trust the news—it is still subject to much more rigorous standards than what you'll find in a Facebook Group or what you'll hear from your friend Bob down at the dive bar.

But when it comes to getting your health information, I encourage you to be on high alert for these biases, motives, and conflicts of interest.

- Who is in charge of telling the health stories you see?

- Who is helped by these stories?

- Who is often left out of these stories?

- And finally, how do your own biases and motivations impact the stories you pay attention to and amplify?

Read the damn article.

I guess this could have been first on the list of how to decode the latest health headlines, but I wanted to give you all the benefit of the doubt. Then I thought, *Eh, better include it just in case.* I promise this has nothing to do with any lack of faith in you. It has everything to do with the fact that this is a trap that even I continue to fall into. I'm busy. And you're busy. We're all really freaking busy. And sometimes we get a push alert to our phones with a headline and we're like, *Great, noted,* before we swipe to dismiss it and go back to whatever we were doing.

But here's what happened in the five seconds it took for you to do that: You absorbed that headline and only that headline. That's what you'll remember when that topic comes up again.

As someone who has written a lot of headlines over the years, I can promise you that they do not contain all the information the reader is meant to know. They can't possibly. A particularly annoying example of this popped out at me while I was writing this very chapter. The headline was: "Experts warn birth-control pills could increase the risk of 'deadly blood clots' in coronavirus patients."[45]

Well, shit, said this writer, a person taking birth control pills and currently living through the coronavirus pandemic. I'm guessing a lot of people had similar reactions.

And then I read the article, in which they state three separate times that "more research is needed" to determine if this is a thing or not. That got me thinking: *What research do they have then?* Unfortunately, this article didn't include a link to the actual research paper anywhere. (A red flag from earlier, if you're keeping score!) But after a little sleuthing I was able to find the actual journal article.[46] And in that paper was this very helpful tidbit, which I certainly would have appreciated reading in the article: "As this Commentary is being submitted, no reports of increased incidence of VTEs in pregnant women or women taking estrogen preparations who also have COVID-19 have emerged."

So basically, there are currently no reports of birth control leading to deadly blood clots in coronavirus patients. What a vastly different headline that would have been!

Obviously I know that we're going to read way more headlines than full articles. That's just a reality. Just remember, though, the way that headlines have a tendency to get stuck in your head and influence everything from your mood to your perception to your anxiety. And remember that they're not the whole story.

Check the date.

If I had a nickel for every "breaking" health story that someone sent me from 2012, I swear...

GROUNDBREAKING TREATMENT? GAME-CHANGING DRUG? HERE'S HOW TO TELL IF YOU SHOULD CARE OR NOT.

Of all the different types of health headlines, these have perhaps the biggest chance of actually helping or harming someone. That's why these health stories are the primary focus of HealthNewsReview.org, a project that does exactly what its name suggests: systematically reviews health news, separating the responsible reporting from the not so much.

A well-known watchdog of health journalism, HealthNewsReview.org was founded in 2006 by career health journalist Gary Schwitzer, and at one time involved a team of over 50 people reviewing health headlines and creating resources to help both journalists and consumers better understand the messages we're exposed to.

"What we based our project on was where the rubber meets the road, and that is to systematically evaluate media messages that make claims about interventions," Schwitzer tells me. "That's where it all starts, whether it is a screening test, a blood test, a diagnostic test, a treatment, a product, a procedure, a lifestyle change—we need to help that patient, that consumer to become smarter and to understand how to evaluate the evidence and improve their own critical thinking before they go in waving an article in the face of their primary care provider."

Schwitzer and his team did that with a list of 10 criteria for evaluating a health news story—with 10 out of 10 being the ideal. They reviewed more than 2,600 health news stories from outlets like the Associated Press, the *New York Times,* Vox, CNN, and BuzzFeed.

I can't remember when I first learned about HealthNewsReview.org, but I sure as hell remember getting reviewed by them. It was one of my last articles at BuzzFeed, an explainer about the female condom, and you guys . . . I GOT A 10 OUT OF 10. I am quite possibly prouder of that than any other professional achievement to date. Seriously. I don't think Schwitzer realized just how much I was fangirling at the fact that I finally got to talk to him while writing this book.

Unfortunately, HealthNewsReview.org lost its funding in 2018. I guess evaluating the validity and usefulness of the health stories we're seeing every day just wasn't something that people with money wanted to invest in. And that's deeply unsettling. The wellness industry is out there thriving, while the watchdogs don't have the funding to continue to tell you what's actually worth your time and money. That sucks.

Misinformation and misleading headlines sure aren't going anywhere, so I hope Schwitzer's project isn't either. But because one watchdog can only do so much, I want to share the 10 criteria that HealthNewsReview.org has used to evaluate thousands of health stories over the years. I hope you'll use them in your own life—whether you're watching a news segment on a groundbreaking new treatment or reading about some new miracle cure on social media.

1. Does the story explain how much this actually costs?

2. Does the story say how effective this is, and are you shown the data to back that up?

3. Does the story also provide information on any potential harms and how likely they are to happen?

④ Does the story explain the quality of the evidence behind this?

⑤ Does the story commit disease-mongering or a misrepresentation of a condition/symptom/risk factor in the interest of selling a solution that people might not actually need?

⑥ Does the story include independent sources and identify any conflicts of interest?

⑦ Does the story explain how this new intervention stacks up against existing alternatives (in price, effectiveness, availability, etc.)?

⑧ Does the story mention if this new treatment is actually available and accessible to you?

⑨ Does the story clearly establish what exactly is new or "groundbreaking" about this?

⑩ Does the whole story seem to rely on a press release for a drug company or medical organization?

How to not fall for the latest wellness trend all over Instagram

WHAT WAS THE LAST WELLNESS PRODUCT YOU BOUGHT OFF the internet that you were just *absolutely sure* was going to change your life? Mine was a cellulite cream for my butt.

It had incredible reviews everywhere I looked. It was packed with natural-sounding ingredients that promised to tighten and smooth. It smelled like summer and not caring that your ass was hanging out of your swimsuit. It was vegan and gluten-free—as if my butt (or my mouth, for that matter) cared about those things. I slathered it all over my body with the confidence of someone who had done their research before they bought it.

It gave me the gnarliest rash. And, you guys . . . I kept using it.

I told myself that maybe something else was causing these tiny itchy bumps to progressively spread from my hamstrings to the rest of my body. I just really, really didn't want it to be the butt cream. I had spent money on this thing. I felt comforted by all of the positive reviews. I liked the way it looked on my nightstand and the way it felt on my skin. I felt a weird sort of loyalty toward it?

Eventually I stopped using it, and the rash promptly dissipated—along with all of my hopes for a cellulite-free behind. And I kept that damn product on my nightstand for over a year . . . not willing to admit defeat and toss it in the trash.

That's what happens when we want so badly for something to work—especially when we've already invested our time and money into it. We end up investing a little bit of our hopes and dreams into it, too.

I share this story not to brag about my cellulite or my very sensitive skin, but to remind you that you're not the only person who falls for a brilliant marketing plan and ends up wildly disappointed at the results—only to go all in on the next tempting wellness fad the following week. I've been there.

> *That's what happens when we want so badly for something to work—especially when we've already invested our time and money into it. We end up investing a little bit of our hopes and dreams into it, too.*

And a cellulite cream that broke me out instead of smoothing me out is hardly the tip of the wellness market iceberg. The stakes were pretty low on that one, I'll admit. Other times, the wellness fads we buy and buy into are propped up on much bigger, loftier health promises. And in those cases, the downfall that occurs when this thing doesn't live up to the hype—or, worse, is actually harmful—is much more damaging.

I've tried and trashed so many health and wellness products over the years. I'm talking immune boosters, probiotic pills, cranberry supplements, CBD balms, various essential oils, charcoal masks, organic tampons, organic protein powder, organic pre-workout, de-bloat tea (definitely be near a bathroom with that one), and so on. Most of this stuff landed on my desk when I was a health editor, and I'm not one to be wasteful. Other things I bought with my own money, because sometimes that branding really just gets you, you know?

I feel like I'm not alone here, right? It's so easy to buy into the promise in the packaging. And it's even easier when you're not necessarily engaging with an advertisement—you're getting actual recommendations from people you actually kind of almost know . . . or at least follow. I'm talking about the bounty of wellness trends and products on social media.

If you're on social media at all, you've probably spotted an influencer posting sponcon about the latest wellness fad that "changed their life!"—whether it's CBD gummies or detox teas or herbal supplements. They might even include phrases like "research-backed" or "scientifically tested" to really seal the deal. And, look, they have a promo code for 20 percent off!

Now, listen, I'm not here to judge how anyone makes money off of their brand or to look down on someone who genuinely tried and liked something. If you want to drink celery water all damn day, you do you! My concern, as always, is when a well-meaning influencer with a massive platform shares health misinformation—especially if that misinformation could cost you money or put your health in jeopardy. That concern is amplified when I consider that many of these fads are far more accessible to people than quality, affordable, compassionate medical care—which means that the people who are harmed most by this will be those who are already underserved by our health care system.

Let's zoom out for a bit and think about why these wellness fads do so well in the first place. It's typically a product or hack that promises to fix an embarrassing or annoying health problem in the comfort of your own home. The whole idea hinges on you acknowledging that something on your body is not normal and needs fixing—whether it's your weight, your skin, your sex drive, your general ass-dragging, whatever. They tell you that you aren't alone for worrying about whatever problem you're worrying about, that no one listened to them either, and that finally—finally!—they found something that helped. Click the link in bio for more.

No one can blame you for wanting a fast and easy fix to something you're stressing about—even if you only started stressing about it five minutes after seeing their post. I've definitely been there. But I've also spent a not-insignificant portion of my career writing and editing debunkers of these "fast fixes." And after about your 20th article on things your vagina doesn't need, you become a bit of an expert on how to be a more conscious consumer of the wellness trends, fads, and products du jour.

All of that reporting taught me how to stay mindful and skeptical when surrounded by a wellness industry that's constantly trying to sell us something to fix our body issues—real or imaginary. Now, I want to help sharpen your own bullshit detector. So here are my ground rules for not falling for the latest wellness trend all over Instagram—or wherever else you're personally attacked with pseudoscience.

Ask yourself: Does this kinda make me feel like shit?

I like to start with this red flag because it can be a subtle one, but it's also pretty damn telling. For me, it's a great way to immediately identify something as not worth your time, money, and energy.

If a product's marketing—or even an influencer's social media post about it—grounds the message in telling you that something on or in your body is wrong/gross/unsightly/embarrassing/not normal/just generally unideal, then keep on scrolling. We don't trust them, we don't respect them, and we sure as hell don't want to give them our money.

Think of it as wellness negging. You've definitely seen this. It's an ad campaign that tells you you'll be so much more confident once you take care of that awkward thing—that you didn't actually feel awkward about before now. It's the influencer who says all bodies are beautiful, but *she* just feels healthiest when *she* does this cleanse six times a year. It's the Instagram ad that implies you can't possibly feel clean after your period unless you're using these scented vaginal wipes. Honestly, only peasants have vaginas that smell like vaginas.

If something simultaneously makes you feel like shit and also like you need to get out your credit card, please stop. Sleep on it. Impulse buy candles and gum—not something to "fix" your body.

Don't trust testimonials over science-based medicine.

I know, I know . . . I'm sure I sound like a broken record by now. But this point really does deserve to be in every chapter of this book, because it's one of the hardest habits for us to break. It's basically asking us to go against our natural impulses. Anecdotal evidence may be some of the weakest science, but it also tends to be the most convincing. We might say we want "just the facts," but we still turn our attention away from a boring list of data in favor of a wild documentary series, an "I Tried It" video on YouTube, or an egregiously long Facebook post from someone you haven't spoken to in 12 years.

Stories are what stick with us—not a list of facts. When your cousin tells you that deodorant caused her breast cancer, that story is going to be hard to shake—even when confronted with the fact that there is absolutely no research proving that deodorant causes breast cancer.[47] Or when your friend swears that these probiotic supplements cured all of her tummy troubles, you're probably going to believe her despite the fact that there is very limited research on the usefulness of probiotic supplements in healthy adults dealing with occasional gut concerns.[48]

It's natural to trust our close spheres of influence—our family, friends, and the people we follow online or in the media—over some big medical organization that you know nothing about or some researchers you've never heard of. You also don't want to be the "well, actually . . ." person when some-one is telling you about their personal experience. Sometimes we don't care about the data and the research—we care about what's happening in our own bodies. We care about what we believe and feel.

So I'm not telling you to go tell Susan that she and her supplements are full of shit. That would be rude. But I'm urging you to make your own health decisions based on definitive data, rather than word of mouth—particularly when those decisions involve you spending money or putting something into your body.

Watch out for fear-based finger-pointing.

Here's another red flag that people often don't realize until I point it out to them. It's a common marketing strategy that you'll find everywhere from commercials and product packaging to influencer posts. It might even slip out in personal recommendations from friends and family members. I call it fear-based finger-pointing.

The most obvious example of this that I can't seem to escape is the hype around all-natural, organic, 100 percent cotton tampons. I started to notice it around 2015. I was getting press releases about newer, better-for-you tampons. I was seeing ads on the subway implying that the regular old grocery store tampon currently inside of me was super shady at best.

The marketing all seemed to say—sometimes subtly, sometimes explicitly—that you couldn't trust what was in the tampons you've been using all these years. Those brands haven't been printing their ingredients on the box. So who knows what havoc they could be wreaking on your delicate vagina?! Who knows what's even in them?! It could be chemicals. It could be toxins. It could be tracking devices. (Okay, they didn't actually suggest that last one, but it's about as alarmist as the rest of their message.)

I decided to dig into this for an article—because obviously. I found out that there was truth to the claim that most tampon companies weren't printing their ingredients on the boxes, but you could usually find them on the brand's website. It was pretty easy for me to call up several companies and confirm the ingredients used in their tampons. It's not like it was classified information—there just was never a requirement for it to be on the box, so they didn't put it there.

What that doesn't mean—even though those ads were implying it—is that tampon companies can just throw a bunch of weird stuff in your tampons and call it a day. Tampons are regulated by the FDA as medical devices, which means that before a new tampon hits the shelves, the manufacturer must put it through an FDA review process that involves submitting their testing and safety data.[49] They also need to assure the FDA that their tampons don't contain certain ingredients anywhere near amounts that have been found to be harmful. For instance, the FDA asks manufacturers to confirm that any bleaching processes they used were free of elemental chlorine, which could lead to dangerous levels of dioxin, an environmental pollutant that the World Health Organization says can have negative health effects at high levels.[50]

So tampon manufacturing wasn't exactly rife with chaos and deception. But that's what it seemed like when you saw any of these advertisements for new, organic, all-cotton tampons. They claimed that you had no idea what chemicals or ingredients were in your tampons. They claimed that only organic cotton should be allowed inside of you.

But here's the thing: There is no research showing that tampons made with regular cotton—or even rayon, another common ingredient in many tampons—are harmful. They have not been shown to be less safe than their organic, all-natural counterparts. So let's all calm the fuck down, okay?

All of that fear-based finger-pointing from Team Organic Cotton Tampon made a lot of people worried about their period products. It's pretty brilliant marketing. ("Don't you want to know what you're putting in your body?" *Um, yeah, obviously!*) Too bad it's not based in actual science.

So I wrote an article at the time, telling readers what their vaginas really thought of their tampons. (In short: they didn't really care.) I explained the FDA's review process and the lack of data pointing to OG tampons as dangerous. I interviewed gynecologists who agreed: your tampon is not killing you. Sure, there may be people who are irritated by typical tampons and want to try an alternative to see if it's gentler—just like some of us are irritated by cellulite creams and others aren't. But for the vast majority of people, the bargain buy you've been using is just fine. Having alternatives is good. Marketing them in fear isn't.

I hit publish.

It wasn't long before a representative from one of the new-tampons-on-the-block called me up at work, wanting to discuss my article. She told me I didn't get what they were doing—they were just trying to empower women to make informed decisions about their bodies.

I kindly told her that I appreciated that mission—and I shared it. But I didn't appreciate them dressing up fearmongering as feminism. I didn't appreciate my friends asking me if they needed to splurge on these more expensive tampons now that they were worried about what's in their old ones—when there is no research to suggest that they need to be scared. I didn't appreciate them giving people with periods a new reason to stress out about their bodies. We have enough. I've had enough. (Of course, I'm sure I didn't say it that flawlessly—we never think of the perfect comeback until after the phone call, right?)

That was five years ago, and as I'm sure you've noticed, these products and this marketing didn't go away. You can see this "we're more transparent"/"you can trust us"/"you know what's in us" messaging all over wellness products, from skin care and hair care to nut milks and cleaning products. I hope you'll call it out the next time you see it. And I hope you'll take a few minutes to find out if there's any legitimate reason to be wary of that thing they're telling you to be wary of. In many cases, there isn't.

Remember that natural does not mean safe.

In my time covering health and wellness, I witnessed a significant shift in the way people wanted to take care of themselves and—as a result—the content they responded to.

In 2011, I worked at a magazine that recommended using a toilet seat cover as facial blotting paper in a pinch. The other writers and I heralded it as the perfect wellness tip—it was hacky, it was easy, it was unexpected, it was something that a reader in Kentucky could do just as easily as a reader in LA. We were constantly trying to brainstorm new ideas that lived up to the toilet-seat-cover hack.

In 2019, I edited an article about natural alternatives to retinol. Sure, retinol is highly researched and highly effective, and it's literally vitamin A. But ugh, isn't there a more natural option?

The wellness scene had changed. We went from not caring what we put in or on our bodies as long as it worked to not wanting to put anything in or on our bodies unless we knew exactly what was in it, if we could pronounce it, and if it was sustainably sourced. I'm not saying this is bad—being an informed consumer is great. But it did seem to result in this halo effect when it comes to the word *natural*.

We assume that if something is natural it can't possibly harm us. It can't come with nasty side effects like antibiotics. It can't do anything but wonders for our bodies. Right?

Hate to burst your bubble, but there are tons of things that are natural and harmful—in small and big doses. Plenty of "natural" ingredients in skin care can cause serious irritation or allergic reactions. Essential oils may be "natural," but some can be poisonous if ingested, while others can cause severe chemical burns when mixed with sunlight. Even certain vitamins can be toxic in large doses. So you can see how easy it would be to overdo it on a

> *Just because something doesn't require a prescription doesn't mean that you shouldn't be wary of putting it on or in your body.*

bunch of different wellness products, with no regard for how they might interact with each other, and suddenly you're not feeling so well.

Just because something doesn't require a prescription doesn't mean that you shouldn't be wary of putting it on or in your body. When in doubt, always ask your doctor or pharmacist about any side effects you should keep in mind when using a product—especially if you have any conditions or are taking any other medications or supplements. If you can't do that, at least do some research on the ingredients themselves, paying particular attention to possible side effects and interactions—and not just drug interactions, but interactions with foods, drinks, and other things you're putting in or around your body.

If something is claiming to be a cure-all, it's probably not.

I've covered a lot of "cure-alls" in my years as a health editor. You know, the latest trendy ingredient that's found in everything and purported to help with everything. This is typically a big ol' red flag for me. There are very few things in life that can make pretty much everything better outside of venting to your mom, jumping in the ocean, or punching a heavy bag for an hour. The first thing you have to ask when faced with a "cure-all" is: Okay, how? How does it cure diabetes naturally? How does it kill cancer cells? How does it burn fat while you sleep? How does it reverse your genes? *How?*

What you're looking for here is documented research on the way the actual cure-all had an effect on the actual health outcome in question. But what you typically get are studies showing that one specific component of that cure-all, when given in unrealistically high doses to rats, had an effect on some measure that's kinda close to the condition we're talking about. Obviously that's not ideal, but it's something. Sometimes all we have is research showing the mechanism of action, or how this cure-all *might* affect the condition. That's not ideal either, but again, sometimes it's useful. Just keep in mind that you are unlikely to see the same results as the lab rats, because you are not a lab rat.

What you really don't want to see is no clear line from point *A* to point *B*. If your question of "how?" is answered with a lot of theories and testimonials but no real science, I'd skip it.

Manage your expectations.

This isn't an exhaustive list of how to avoid spending money on wellness bullshit online. That would be a much bigger book. But the truth is that there isn't really a foolproof plan for knowing if something is worth your time, money, and energy or knowing if something is definitively going to work for you— because bodies are super weird and variable.

That's where peer-reviewed research and FDA regulation come in. I know the process is not perfect and there are always limitations, but the more rigorous research we do on something, the more confident we can be that we understand how it might impact all sorts of people. This is especially important when we're talking about treating conditions, because when you're chronically ill you often don't have the time, money, or energy to waste on treatments that haven't been studied.

That said, just because something hasn't been extensively studied or FDA-approved doesn't mean that it *can't* work. It just means that it hasn't been *proven* to work, nor has it been proven to be *safe*.

You don't need to limit yourself to only partaking in health and wellness things that are rigorously tested and approved. We can just do things because they feel good, because they work for us, because we want to experiment. That's allowed. To my knowledge, no one is working on the FDA approval of laying on the beach as a proven treatment for anxiety, but it sure as hell helps mine and I'm going to keep doing it.

All I ask is that you see the very crucial difference between things that have been through that rigorous process and things that haven't. See that it's irresponsible to make claims or a profit off of something that you swear will make someone healthier, when you don't have the science to back it up. Realize the hypocrisy of someone who tells you to shun the medical researchers who have dedicated their lives to studying something—and asks you to trust them instead. Stay mindful and skeptical, especially when it concerns your health.

> *Realize the hypocrisy of someone who tells you to shun the medical researchers who have dedicated their lives to studying something—and asks you to trust them instead.*

We're all a little bit different. What helps one person may hurt another. What calms one person might stress out another. Even if a hundred people tried the same supplement, you'd expect to see a little bit of variation in the results.

One person's miracle cellulite cream is another person's ass rash.

CHAPTER

How to tackle a health question like a health editor

LET ME TELL YOU ABOUT THE TIME I THOUGHT I WAS GOING BLIND.

I was on a flight to Vegas with my friend, watching Netflix on my phone, minding my own business. Suddenly, there was a big, weird spot in my vision—like that temporary orb you see when you accidentally look right at a light bulb. But I didn't remember looking into any lights . . . and it wasn't going away. I blinked a few times. Still there. I closed my eyes for 10 seconds. Still there. I got up, went to the bathroom, and rubbed my eyes a bit. Still there.

This is when I started to panic. Did I somehow look out the window and catch a glimpse of the literal sun, which at this elevation burned a hole through my retina?! Was this some kind of vision degeneration linked to an underlying condition I didn't know I had? I hadn't been to an eye doctor in decades, ever since they told me I had perfect vision. Should I have been going all along, just in case? I ran through a mental list of things I'd reported on that were associated with vision changes. As you can probably guess, that did nothing for my anxiety.

After we checked into our hotel, I got in the shower and continued to alternate between resting my eyes and blinking incessantly to check whether this weird spot was still there. Over the next several hours, I tried everything to figure it out—to confirm its existence and prove I wasn't just seeing things. I noticed it most when I opened and closed my eyes, but it was also clearly visible in my line of sight, like a blurry smudge obstructing my view. When I closed my right eye to put on eyeliner, it was clear that the smudge was just in my left eye—not both. What the fuck was happening to me?

I decided not to tell my friend, knowing that I would probably sound ridiculous, not to mention it would make it much harder to try to ignore this and hope it would go away.

It's probably nothing, I told myself over and over again. *It'll go away.*

But it didn't go away.

A full month went by before I sought help. (There goes that care-avoidant health anxiety again, I guess.) And in that month, I fought the urge every single day to type my symptoms into Google. I knew myself, and I knew Google. And while I sure as hell didn't know what was going on with my eye, I did know that it wasn't getting worse, I wasn't in pain, and it wasn't severely interfering with my life. I knew I was going to seek out help as soon as the time was right—while I was in Vegas wasn't it, nor was when I was traveling for the holidays. So what would searching my symptoms really change?

It probably wouldn't give me a concrete answer. And it probably *would* give me more to be anxious about. It definitely wouldn't change the fact that I already knew I needed to talk to a medical professional about this—not a search engine.

Still, I was freaking out. And I was frustrated at myself for freaking out. How could I be so calm and confident when it came to reporting on health issues—prioritizing facts and data—and yet still assume the worst was out to get my own body? Why couldn't I listen to logic and reason the same way I hoped my readers would?

Eventually, something clicked. It was like getting slapped in the face with a mix of self-awareness and almost a decade's worth of health reporting experience. Maybe I *could* tackle my own health concerns like a health editor. I mean, why not try?

So I started where I always start when reporting a health article—finding the experts. Where would I go if I were reporting on a rare, scary vision issue plaguing a generally healthy 30-year-old woman? I would start with an academic hospital—where the physicians aren't just treating patients but are also conducting research on a regular basis. After some digging, I found that NYU Langone Eye Center is not only an academic health facility, but also one that conducts research specifically on conditions affecting the retina. Bingo. Then I scrolled through a bunch of physician profiles until I found someone whose research background seemed particularly interesting. Book appointment.

It should be noted here in big bold letters **the immense privilege** I have that put me in a position to do all that. I was employed, insured, living in a city where this renowned teaching hospital was just a subway stop away, and I was reasonably certain I could afford whatever medical care awaited me. But in addition to that, I knew where and how to look for that care.

After several stressful vision tests—only stressful because I hadn't been to an eye doctor in so long and was thoroughly unsettled by every contraption that I was asked to stick my face into—the doctor came into the room and said she had good news and bad news. The good news was that I wasn't going blind—nor was I dealing with some progressive vision problem that was tied to some unknown illness. The bad news was that this smudge in my eye wasn't going to go away.

She diagnosed me with something called acute macular neuroretinopathy. When you do Google it—as I finally allowed myself to do once I got home from the appointment—one of the first things you'll see is this definition: "Acute macular neuroretinopathy (AMN) is a rare disease of unknown etiology that most commonly affects young to middle-aged females."[51] (FYI: "Unknown etiology" means they don't really know what causes this.)

Apparently this condition wasn't even described in medical literature until 1975, and it's still considered pretty rare. It turns out that advanced imaging techniques like those contraptions I was asked to stick my head into are finally allowing doctors to better diagnose it, understand it, and study it. According to a comprehensive review of the literature in 2016, which still only looked at 101 cases of AMN, the typical patient is female, white, and in their thirties (check, check, check).[52] There's no known cause, but there are a few potential risk factors that stand out among the research, including a recent flu-like illness, oral contraceptive use, exposure to epinephrine or ephedrine, and recent trauma. Caffeine consumption was also noted as a possible risk factor.

While I 100% fit the demographic profile, the only risk factors I seemed to check off were using birth control pills and being in a strong, committed relationship with coffee. But the specialist I saw said she wasn't concerned enough to tell me to quit birth control or caffeine—the research just wasn't sufficient to say that either of those things actually caused this weird little dot in my vision.

Well, if you believe in the power of manifestation, I had finally done it. I ended up with a rare health issue with no known cause. But . . . I'm okay. Seriously, I'm fine. And I can see perfectly fine, too. As the ophthalmologist assured me on that first visit, my eyes adjusted to this weird smudge, and pretty soon I barely noticed it. I can still see it in my line of vision when I close my right eye, but I don't notice it on a daily basis anymore. More importantly, it's not something that causes panic to swell inside of me, sure that it's a sign of something serious and seriously terrifying.

I realize that this could have gone very differently. I could have been given a diagnosis that would forever change my life in scary, costly ways. I still might. We all might. But at some point we have to learn to live with that certain uncertainty. I'm not going to lie and say I'm totally there, but I'm starting to entertain the idea.

For me, at least, the hardest part is separating what I *think* and *feel* from what I *know*—from what the data shows us and from what is logical. This, I've realized, is the reason why I could be an award-winning health journalist as well as someone who spends an uncomfortable amount of time worrying about carbon monoxide poisoning and blood clots. My health editor hat compels me to work from a place of logic, reason, and skepticism. But when it's off, I can quickly convince myself that I could very well be the 1 person out of 100,000 to die from a certain illness . . . despite not having any of the symptoms or risk factors.

That's why I don't want you to feel embarrassed or silly or uninformed when you fall victim to an all-too-tempting wellness fad or when you spend a ridiculous amount of time, money, and energy searching for a way to feel better. It is very hard to think logically and objectively when it's your own body you're worrying about. Trust me, I know.

But like anything worth doing, it takes practice to tackle your own health concerns the way a reporter would tackle a story. Hell, even a seasoned health reporter has trouble with it. After quite a bit of trial and error, I created a kind of personal guidebook for doing just that, drawing on a lot of the same tools I use when working out the details of a complicated article. The tips in this chapter are the same tips I tell myself when I'm going through it. My suggestion is to read through the following steps before you really need them, and then maybe bookmark this for the next time you're freaking out about a health concern.

First, know when *not* to Google.

Let's start with the biggest hurdle, shall we? When you have a health concern, your first inclination is typically to consult the internet. And as I covered in chapter 2, there are a lot of very valid reasons why we do this. But remember the main one, especially for people who experience health anxiety: to seek reassurance and rid ourselves of uncertainty.

But when, in all of your years of symptom searching, has asking Dr. Google ever truly eliminated your uncertainty? It sure as hell hasn't ever left me feeling warm, fuzzy, and fully healed. Don't get me wrong, there are a lot of great health information and solid resources online, but you have to know where to look and what to ask. And when we're freaking out about our bodies, we're often not yet in the right headspace for that.

So how do you know if it's a smart, safe idea to consult the internet with a health concern? I'd ask yourself the following question first: what do you hope to gain from this search?

> *So how do you know if it's a smart, safe idea to consult the internet with a health concern? I'd ask yourself the following question first: what do you hope to gain from this search?*

Now, be honest. Are you primarily seeking reassurance? Are you looking for some big flashing sign that you are either totally fine or totally dying? If that's your goal—to eliminate as much uncertainty as possible—remember that the internet will almost never be able to offer you that peace of mind. And it's not because of a lack of reputable information. It's because when we're in this reassurance-seeking mindset, no amount of information on the internet will satisfy our appetite for answers.

A perfect example of this is the story I told before about my abnormal Pap smear result that led me to search in a panic for information—eventually landing on an article I had written on the very topic. I told myself I was trying to arm myself with as much information as possible to feel more prepared for my biopsy. But that was a lie. I was looking for reassurance. I was looking for answers that didn't exist—not online and not even on the other end of the phone with my doctor. She wasn't withholding information from me. I was just at a point in that particular health journey where we were awaiting answers. And no amount of wandering around online was going to take away that uncertainty.

That's not to say that the information out there wasn't helpful. (I like to think that the many articles I wrote and edited about abnormal Pap test results were very informative.) But they just don't come with guarantees. So stop and ask yourself what you're really searching for. If it's just a little extra information to make you feel more prepared and empowered—have at it. But if you know that what you really want is certainty in a time of stressful uncertainty, remind yourself that you aren't likely to find it on the other end of the search results.

Instead, try to sit with that uncertainty. Go back to chapter 4 and try putting your thoughts on trial. Maybe institute the 24-hour rule. Turn off your Wi-Fi. Sometimes giving ourselves some time and space helps us see our concerns with a little more objectivity. And if after a brief time-out you're still craving information or resources that the internet can reasonably provide, you have my permission to start searching. But before you do, make sure you know what you're really asking. Which brings me to the next step . . .

Narrow your focus.

I don't know about you, but I have a tendency to spiral when it comes to health and body questions. My concern is very rarely something specific and concrete. Instead it's usually a question tangled up in several other worries, buried at the bottom of a pit of existential dread. Basically it's that big mess of earbuds and necklaces at the bottom of your purse that gives you anxiety every time you look at it or even think about it.

> *You need to pluck out the one true question at the source of your anxiety spiral before you can expect to find solutions.*

In case you haven't noticed, this kind of snowballing of concerns is not very conducive to getting answers. You need to pluck out the one true question at the source of your anxiety spiral before you can expect to find solutions.

I'll give you an example from recent memory/panic. In the midst of the coronavirus pandemic, I—like many others, I imagine—entertained the idea on more than one occasion that I definitely had it. One particularly memorable time was in May 2020, when I made the very stressful but very careful decision to rent a car and drive to an empty lake house outside of New York City with my friend and her husband for a week. We had all spent the previous two months taking every precaution, which made this trip equally terrifying and satisfying.

We spent our days working from our laptops in various sun-drenched corners of the house, which seemed sprawling compared to our tiny apartments, then logged off and hopped into kayaks before making dinner. It was the most sun and social interaction I had had in months. It was amazing. And then I noticed a rash.

I realize that a skin rash is a very rare symptom of COVID-19. I had seen the headlines. And it would be just my luck that I would get one of those rare symptoms . . . or at least that's what my health anxiety was telling me. And now I had a rash of very tiny red bumps on the front of my throat. It didn't itch or burn. It was just there—taunting me every time I looked in the mirror, making me question every decision I had made.

Do you know how hard it was not to Google "coronavirus rash" and scroll through articles for hours, comparing them to my neck in the mirror? IT WAS SO HARD. Then, of course, I started becoming hypervigilant about any other possible symptoms. I felt hot and achy. I had a sore throat. This was for sure coronavirus, right?

I willed myself to put my phone down and breathe. I reminded myself to think like a health reporter. What was I actually asking? *Do I have coronavirus?* No, no, it needs to be more specific than that. *Is this particular constellation of symptoms—a rash, sore throat, and feeling feverish—a sign of coronavirus?* I mean, MAYBE?!

So I put my thoughts on trial: Do I actually have all of these symptoms? My temperature was normal. (Yes, of course I had brought a thermometer with me.) I was most likely feeling hot because it was 83 degrees in my bedroom and I didn't have an air conditioner. My sore throat was most likely due to the massive amounts of pollen covering everything in sight—same as every year. And I was only achy in the muscles I used to kayak—the same muscles I hadn't used in months. So really, my question came down to the rash. *Is this rash a rare sign of coronavirus or something else?*

I instituted the 24-hour rule, promising myself I would try to go to sleep, and if I was still wondering about this question the next day, I would let myself search it out and decide what to tell my friends. When I woke up the next morning, the rash—most likely a heat rash—was gone.

Of course, there have also been times when the 24-hour rule didn't end in such a quick, clean resolution. There have been times when symptoms were still there—even instances when they got progressively worse. But that time-out can be crucial to narrowing your focus.

When you're freaking out about something going on with your body and you want answers, the first step is making sure your question is specific and clear. If this feels unfair—that you would be expected to be articulate and precise at a time when you're panicking about your health—you're right, it is unfair. But it's also, unfortunately, necessary. Think about the first question a doctor or nurse asks you when they open the exam room door.

○ **"What brought you in today?"**

○ **"What's bothering you?"**

○ **"What can I help you with?"**

I realize that you're not in front of a doctor or nurse yet. You might be in front of your computer or in front of your bathroom mirror, thoughts spiraling with a million questions and worst-case scenarios. In that moment, my advice to you is this: Pause. Take a deep breath in and out. And try to sum up your chief complaint or concern in one question.

Let's use an example many of us can relate to: wondering why the hell your period is so weird. It's a valid question, but it's also incredibly broad. Simply asking the internet or a medical provider if your period is "normal" won't likely address your exact concerns. Can you drill down into what *specifically* it is about your period that seems off?

If you need some examples of what that looks like, I dug into the search data and found a few of the most common period-related queries:

1 Spotting before period

2 Period blood clots

3 Brown period blood

4 Period cramps

5 Irregular periods

All highly relatable, right? If you've ever wondered about one of those things, you are definitely not alone. But even within each of these more specific period searches, there is so much room for variability. What *you* mean by period cramps might be totally different from what *I* mean by period cramps. The type of spotting *you're* talking about might be totally different from the spotting *I'm* talking about.

Try to get even more specific. That might look like:

○ Why do I see a little bit of blood when I wipe even when I'm two weeks out from my period?

○ Why do I sometimes pass these gnarly, dime-sized clots of blood—usually on the second day of my period?

○ Why is my blood a terrifying shade of brown at the beginning and end of my period?

○ Why are my cramps so bad that I'm basically hunched in the fetal position for days before my period?

○ Why is my period sometimes three days, sometimes seven days and decides to just show up whenever the hell it pleases?

I know that it's hard to distill your concerns into one specific question when your mind is racing with possibilities and your whole body is vibrating with confirmation biases. But doing so will allow you to narrow your focus in order to think and act more clearly—whether your next move is to type that question into your phone, call your physician, or pray that your symptoms resolve themselves in the morning. The first step is making sure you know what you're asking—whether you're concerned about your period, your skin, your bowel movements, or the bumpy texture of your breasts.

In fact, I suggest physically writing out your question on a piece of paper. (You can also type it out in the notes app in your phone if that's easier.) There's power in getting those thoughts out of your head and into the world. Once you've written it down, you can read back those words with a little more distance and perspective. Think of it as a low-lift, low-risk way to practice voicing your concerns—something that will only benefit you when it comes time to see a medical professional.

You might find that this actually feels really hard to do. If you start experiencing a little hesitation, a little embarrassment, a little shame, a little fear—take note of that. That's important. Honestly, it's reasonable, given everything we know and don't know about our bodies. That hesitation is the same hesitation that keeps us from speaking up when something feels off. That embarrassment is what stops us from asking questions when we don't understand. That shame is what tells us it's "inappropriate" to talk about our bodies. That fear is what's preventing us from seeking help.

Recognize how much power exists in simply articulating your specific questions and concerns about your health. That's the same power I felt every time I started getting somewhere with a health article. It's scary to ask the hard questions, unsure of the answers you're going to get, but how great is it to not let fear hold you back from seeking solutions?

Find the experts.

Once you know what you're asking, it's time to find out where to do the asking. As I've said, this is by far the most valuable skill I cultivated as a health reporter. And it's also a skill that I firmly believe everyone can develop.

In chapter 5, I taught you how to find trustworthy sources for health information. And if we're tackling our concerns like a health editor, then those same strategies apply.

Knowing the right experts will help you to search smarter. Rather than looking for just your question and leaving it up to the algorithm to tell you what to read, start by searching for your question + the source you trust on this topic.

For example, if I have a question about an abnormal Pap result, I would want to know what the National Cancer Institute has to tell me about that—because the Pap test looks for changes that might signal cervical cancer. So instead of just typing in "abnormal Pap result," I would type in "abnormal Pap result National Cancer Institute," and those search results would be much more helpful. In fact, the first link should take you to a comprehensive guide to understanding abnormal Pap results and what comes next. See how much easier that was?

That said, you probably don't always know what source to type into the search bar alongside your concern. To help with that, I've put together the following list of sources that I go back to time and again—whether I'm reporting on an issue or wondering about it myself. This is by no means exhaustive, but it's a good place to start.

COMMON HEALTH CONCERNS AND CURIOSITIES	MY GO-TO SOURCE (OR SOURCES)
Anything involving the vagina, uterus, and related reproductive organs (whether you're interested in reproducing or not)	American College of Obstetricians and Gynecologists (ACOG)
Skin, hair, and nails	American Academy of Dermatology
Cancer	National Cancer Institute, American Cancer Society

Birth control	Bedsider, Planned Parenthood, ACOG
Gut and butt stuff, diabetes, and kidney issues	National Institute of Diabetes and Digestive and Kidney Diseases
Allergies, asthma, and infectious diseases	National Institute of Allergy and Infectious Diseases
Mental health	National Institute of Mental Health, American Psychiatric Association, American Psychological Association
Sleep questions	National Sleep Foundation
Intel on medications, medical procedures, and medical devices	Food and Drug Administration (FDA)
Stats and facts about various diseases and conditions	Centers for Disease Control and Prevention (CDC)
Health screening recommendations	U.S. Preventive Services Task Force (USPSTF)
Mouth, teeth, and gum stuff	American Dental Association
General health information on a broad range of topics	MedlinePlus (which is run by the National Library of Medicine)

Another smart way to find legitimate, expert-backed information on a particular health topic is to look for academic medical centers in the search results. These are teaching hospitals—like Johns Hopkins, Mayo Clinic, NYU Langone—that also typically have super helpful websites covering the topics that their staff encounter every day. Their websites also usually let you browse through their research and their physicians, which is a great way to find a specialist with experience treating and studying the exact topic you're interested in.

There's a big difference between searching for "endometriosis treatments" and "endometriosis treatments academic hospital." The former will give you a ton of great information on treatment options for endometriosis, but the latter will give you the same information from teaching hospitals that diagnose, treat, and research this topic on a regular basis. The fact is that you can find just about anything on the internet, so why settle for casting a super-wide net when you could instead be really specific and still get thousands—if not millions—of results?

HOT TIP: BE A DOMAIN SNOB SOMETIMES

To be honest, I went back and forth a few times about including this tip, but eventually, I decided that the potential benefit to you was worth ruffling a few feathers. So here we are. As a former health reporter, I know the value of rigorously reported health journalism—the kind that typically lives at a link that ends in .com. Quality health reporting has the ability to dig deep and paint a picture of the breadth of research on a topic—including all the controversies and unanswered questions that you might not be privy to if you simply listened to one expert at one medical organization.

But sometimes, you don't have time for nuance, commentary, or compelling anecdotes. Maybe you know exactly what you're looking for, like the prevalence of colorectal cancer in someone your age. Or maybe you don't know what you're looking for, but you know you want to avoid going down a rabbit hole of reporting that might just make you more confused and anxious.

In times like those, there's a simple way to pare down your search results: Opt for sites that end in .org or .gov rather than .com. A .org tells you you're dealing with an organization or nonprofit, while a .gov is reserved for government organizations. For instance, the websites for the CDC and the FDA are hosted on .gov domains, while organizations like the Mayo Clinic and the American Academy of Dermatology have sites hosted on .org domains.

The thing is, there's no guarantee that everything you read on these websites is accurate, up to date, and the *most* authoritative; in fact, as a health reporter I often stumbled upon outdated statistics and treatment protocols on sites with .org and .gov domains. But if you're hoping to weed out some noise and just get a simple, straightforward answer from a most likely trustworthy source, this is a good tactic to try.

Read through the medical research like a pro.

If you really want to tackle a health question like a health editor, you'll want to get comfortable reading through scholarly journal articles. If you're not familiar with these, a journal article refers to research published in a peer-reviewed journal, like the *Journal of the American Medical Association (JAMA)* or the *Journal of Sexual Medicine*. When you see headlines that make big claims like "New Study Says Ice Cream Makes People Happier," chances are they're reporting on a journal article.

My general rule for whenever you read about a new study or hear about "groundbreaking findings" is this: don't make any moves without reading the research yourself.

I realize that's a pretty big ask, because we're all busy and those papers are dense as hell. But isn't that even more reason to do your due diligence? Don't you want to see the receipts before you spend your time, money, or energy on this latest thing?

A FEW TIMES WHEN JOURNAL ARTICLES COME IN HANDY

- When a new medication is approved for a condition you have and you want to see how it stacks up against your current medication

- Before you spend an obscene amount of money on a skin care product with a trendy new ingredient that's supposed to solve all your skin issues

- When a headline seems a little too good to be true (I'm looking at you, "Tequila Helps You Lose Weight, Says Science"!)

- When you hear rave reviews about a certain supplement and you want to know if there's any legitimate science to back it up

I'm not saying that reading peer-reviewed research needs to become your new favorite pastime. But knowing how to find and read these studies can be really empowering. I can't tell you how proud I was when my sister emailed me a few questions about a peer-reviewed study she had found that related to a treatment method her doctor had suggested. It turns out there was some conflicting research on the protocol that was suggested to her, so we each read through the research and came up with a list of questions to ask her doctor to get more clarity on the recommendation. That's the kind of informed, collaborative care I love to see.

So if you're ready to get more comfortable reading through medical research when necessary, here are a few ground rules that will help:

○ **Know how to find research on the topic you're interested in.** One easy way to do this is to go to Scholar.Google.com, which basically limits your Google search to just scholarly articles. Then you can search for things like "birth control and depression" to see a list of scholarly articles related to that topic. From there, you can filter by publish date, which is a helpful way to see the most recent research on a given topic—because things do change! Another great resource for finding studies is PubMed, which allows you to filter by publish date as well as the type of journal article and how much of it you'll be able to access for free.

○ **Read more than just the study abstract.** The abstract of the study is essentially the TL;DR version. It's also free, whereas the full text of a study might be behind a paywall. But the abstract leaves out tons of important information that can totally change the takeaway for the average person. Also, I've definitely found typos in study abstracts that were pretty freaking crucial in reporting on the results. If all you can find is an abstract, try copying and pasting the title of the article into your search engine and seeing if the full text is available for free on another site. If not, your options are either pay for full access or email the corresponding author (there will be an email listed in the Author Affiliations) to see if they might send you a copy. Pro Tip: If you're a college student, you can typically get access through your school's library.

○ **Read the whole damn thing, but especially the Methods and Results sections.** Honestly, the whole paper is important, but if you're strapped for time and just want to know (1) what the study found, and (2) if it applies to you, then these are the main sections you'll be interested in. The Methods section tells you who and what the researchers studied. This is key to understanding if the results actually apply to you or not. The Methods section will tell you if they were working with a nationally representative sample of 10,000 people or if they looked at lab rats, organisms in a petri dish, or 12 white male college students. That matters! The Methods section will also tell you how they studied something. For instance, did they randomly assign two groups to get either a placebo or a medication—and no one involved knew who got what until the study was finished? Or did they just ask people to fill out a survey about which medications they took in the past? Knowing the way a study was conducted can help you understand what limitations might exist.

Then comes the Results section, which tells you what they found. Again, it's usually not as simple as "this caused that!" so read it carefully. Did they find correlation or causation? Did they control for other random variables that might have played a role? For more clarity on what the researchers suggest doing with these results, make sure to read the Discussion section.

Don't try to do it all alone.

There were a lot of times when I was reporting a complicated health story that I just hit a wall. I did my interviews, I compiled my research, I had tons of information. Then I had to write the damn thing, and it all felt so big and overwhelming. I didn't know where or how to start. And each time that happened, the solution was simple: talking it out.

One of the most valuable and validating parts of being a health reporter is talking out a story with another editor—going over my findings, telling them about the big insights I was most energized about, and sharing with them where I was stuck. We dig ourselves into a hole sometimes when we dive deep into a topic. We need to share our findings, questions, and concerns with another person to fully grasp what we learned and what to actually do with this information.

The same is true when you're tackling your own health question.

Doing your own research is important, but I don't want to give the illusion here that you can or should solve your health problems at home. All of these tools and tips are meant to get you to a place where you are more informed, empowered, confident, and capable—no matter what your concern is. Once you've reached that stage, it's time to talk with someone who can help.

Hey, you. You got this.

I had the unfortunate opportunity of putting this chapter into practice recently when I had a health scare just as I was finishing up the book. It started with concerning test results, followed by some very painful procedures, followed by a lot of pacing and waiting for answers. When I finally got the results of the biopsies, I had to laugh. I'm paraphrasing here, but basically the doctor told me: *It's probably nothing. But it could be something. Let's keep an eye on it.*

Folks, there will always be uncertainty about our health. No amount of tips or tricks from me is going to change that. But hopefully, when you're faced with that uncertainty, you don't feel helpless. Hopefully you can use these tactics to feel a little more informed, a little more prepared, a little more confident, a little more capable.

You got this.

How to get the inclusive, empathetic, evidence-based care you deserve

OVER THE PAST WEEK, I RACKED UP 18 CALLS IN TOTAL TO MY health care provider, pharmacy, and insurance company trying to refill a routine prescription that I've been on for years. It started with my new insurance company telling me I needed something called "prior authorization" from my provider, which apparently wasn't the same as . . . the prescription they gave me for this medication. So I called my provider to request that, and I was told a day later that my insurance company rejected it. Cool, cool.

I called my provider again to ask them to make an appeal, and they assured me they would. I waited a few days to be polite before pestering them about that appeal, then finding out they still hadn't done it. So I called my insurance company to ask why, exactly, they weren't approving my medication and what specific words they needed to hear from my provider in order to change their minds. Then I called back my provider, relaying that message and the telephone number they needed to call in order to get this show on the road.

The next day, I got word that the medication was approved, so I called the pharmacy back to ask them to run it again—this time it should be covered. They told me it was covered, but it would still be $305, and they couldn't tell me why. After another call to my insurance company, I eventually discovered that I hadn't yet met my deductible for prescriptions, which was why the cost was so high this time. Unfortunately, there was no generic option for this medication, but I found on their website that there's a coupon you can ask your pharmacy to apply. I made another call to my pharmacy, had them apply the coupon, and eventually paid $50 to get my damn rosacea medication—the same medication that had been free for years under my previous insurance.

To be clear, I'm not complaining. I have insurance. I have the ability to sit on hold for 47 minutes—multiple times—during the workday without being fired. I have somehow cultivated enough inner strength to not throw my phone out the window when the call drops just as I am connected to a human. I have a provider who acted on my behalf—albeit after several annoying phone calls. I don't have to worry about facing a language barrier, discrimination, or stigma based on any aspect of my identity when I make these calls. And most of all, I have the experience and understanding to patiently and persistently navigate this shitshow when I need to. Make no mistake: Having health insurance is not the only privilege when it comes to health care.

But why, when I carry so much privilege in this scenario, is it still so hard?

> *Make no mistake: Having health insurance is not the only privilege when it comes to health care.*

If you, like me, find it outrageously frustrating to find a doctor who takes your insurance, is close-ish to your job or home, and has availability that even remotely works with your schedule, I hope you'll pause for a moment and recognize the incredible privilege in that scenario. You are already in a better position to get care than so many others, and yet it's still so freaking difficult.

On the other hand, if you struggle to access or afford health care for any number of reasons, I hope you'll pause for a moment and recognize that it isn't your fault that this is so hard. You are trying to work within a system that wasn't built to properly serve you. The burden should not be on you to find inclusive, empathetic, accessible care. But, unfortunately, it is.

No wonder we go searching for wellness fads, fast fixes, and miracle cures. Taking care of yourself shouldn't be this hard.

Listen, I can't solve the health care crisis. I can't break down the many (many!) barriers standing in the way of health equity—the systemic racism, ableism, weight stigma, classism, and unchecked biases that don't go away just because someone puts on a white coat. Achieving health equity will require systemic, structural changes at many levels. I don't want to imply here that the burden is on you, the patient, to figure this out. But I also know that you can't sit around and wait for everything to be figured out either—especially not when you need care today.

So while I can't fix the system, I can offer some assistance and advice from my little corner of the wellness industry—where I've had access to leading public health experts, mountains of medical research, and an endless parade of wellness trends passing by my desk. And from this corner, maybe I can make the process of getting care for a health concern suck just a little bit less. If I could do that—if I could make this unnecessarily complicated process a little bit easier, if I could convince you that you don't have to settle for doctors who are dismissive or discriminatory, if I could point you to resources that might actually be able to give you care that's affordable, empathic, and evidence-based—wow that would be something.

My goal with these final takeaways is to help you take better care of yourself—even and especially when it's all too overwhelming. That's usually when you need help the most.

If you're going to spend money on a wellness hack, let it be this one.

What if I told you there were an amazing health hack that can add years to your life, is evidence-based, and doctors actually swear by it? Sure, it costs money and requires a bit of work, but . . . so do all those other wellness fads you've tried over the years.

Okay, ready for the hack?

It's basic preventive care. It's getting a physical every once in a while, getting your flu shot each year, and getting the recommended health screenings at the recommended times.

I know, it's not very sexy or trendy or fun. It's also unfortunately and frustratingly inaccessible to huge swaths of people. But if you're someone who's constantly looking for the next best way to be healthy, I'd be remiss if I didn't state the obvious—because we're usually really great at ignoring the obvious.

Most of us tend to only interact with the health care system when something is broken or bleeding. The rest of the time, we "do wellness" by going to the gym, buying all-organic products, drinking green juice, and occasionally wondering if we should cleanse or detox some part of our bodies. What does it say about us—and our health care system—that we seem more interested in chugging the juice of a celery stalk every morning than in getting a lifesaving medical screening every once in a while? Folks, there are a lot of wellness scams out there, but preventive care isn't one of them.

That said, I realize there are a lot of reasons why you might avoid medical care. Maybe it's costly and inconvenient. Maybe needles terrify you (same). Maybe you're sick of being stigmatized and discriminated against for your weight, your sexuality, your gender identity, your race, your culture, or something else every time you go to a doctor's office. Maybe you've had one too many doctors tell you, "It's just stress . . . try yoga." Maybe you have a personal or generational history of trauma associated with the medical industry that deters you from seeking help. Maybe you have care-avoidant illness anxiety disorder like your girl here. Maybe you just have no idea where to start.

Whatever your reason or reasons, I hear you, and I acknowledge that your reasons are valid. But I also know that you still deserve good care and good health. And routine preventive care—like getting the vaccines and screening tests recommended for people like you—can help catch and even prevent health issues so that they don't become something bigger and more difficult—not to mention more expensive—to treat. I mean, that's one hell of a wellness hack.

If you need some reminders of why preventive care is so important, here are just a few:

- **Getting a flu shot significantly lowers your risk of dying from the flu.** A 2017 study of adults hospitalized with the flu during the 2013–2014 flu season found that people who had been vaccinated were 52 to 79 percent less likely to die than people who hadn't gotten the flu shot that year.[53]

- **Early detection of breast cancer can give you a broader range of treatment options—including less invasive ones.** Unfortunately, data from 2015 found that only 31 percent of uninsured women in the United States between the ages of 40 and 64 years old got a mammogram in the previous two years, compared with 68 percent of insured women in the same age group.[54]

- **The five-year survival rate for cervical cancer is 92 percent when caught early,**[55] yet over half of cervical cancer cases are caught later than that, typically in people who haven't had a recent Pap smear.[56]

- **The most effective way to prevent colorectal cancer is by screening for precancerous polyps so they can be removed before they turn into cancer. And when colorectal cancer is diagnosed, it's easier to treat the earlier it's caught.**[57] But in 2015, only 63 percent of people in the United States aged 50 and older were up to date on their colorectal cancer screening. When looking at people without insurance, that number dropped to just 25 percent of people.[58]

- **High blood pressure was a primary or contributing cause of death for nearly half a million people in the United States in 2018;**[59] yet many people have no idea what their blood pressure is.

So if you're someone who often spends a lot of time, money, and energy on things meant to get you healthier, I'm going to make one final plea with you to start with the basics.

Before shelling out for bespoke vitamins and supplements, schedule a physical exam. Before going on a cleanse, see if you're getting the recommended amount of fiber in your diet. (Most people aren't.) Before sticking a jade egg into your vagina, make sure you're up to date on your Pap smear and STD tests. Before trying some immune-boosting hack you saw on Instagram, get your damn flu shot.

I'm willing to bet that if we redirected all the time and energy we spend on wellness fads toward preventive care, we might be just a little bit healthier—or, at the very least, more prepared to deal with most health concerns as they come up.

Search for a doctor like you search for tacos—or something else you care deeply about.

I don't buy anything—sheets, towels, bodywash, headphones, flights, whatever—without reading an obnoxious amount of reviews and research first. It annoys my friends and family to no end, but it's my method.

To be clear, it's not a method I would actually suggest for everyday purchases, because it's really fucking time-consuming. But I'm sure there's something in your life that you did that level of rigorous research for, too. Maybe it was your wedding venue, your couch, or your dog. Maybe it was a trip you took. Or maybe it was tacos the last time you were craving Mexican food and really wanted to make sure that you were ordering from a place that was going to rock your world. No judgment, tacos are important.

Whatever it is that you obsessively research before making a decision on, I want you to apply that same methodology to finding a care team. I'm using the term *care team* instead of doctor here, because it's my opinion that inclusive, empathetic, accessible health care doesn't always have to look or feel one certain way. That ingrained assumption, I think, is one reason why people turn away from traditional medical care. But it doesn't have to be that way. My primary care provider sports a man bun, not a tie. My dermatologist is a PA (physician assistant), not an MD. I get my STD screenings done at walk-in clinics just as often as I do in a gynecologist's office. And most of the time when I'm feeling sick, I use a telemedicine app instead of dragging my sick ass to a doctor's office.

Basically, I want you to get care whatever way feels safe and accessible to you. Taking care

> *Basically, I want you to get care whatever way feels safe and accessible to you.*

of your health is going to be so much easier if you feel comfortable, secure, and, you know, *cared* for. Getting medical care—not to mention mental health care—is often a very vulnerable experience. In most cases, the more open and honest you are, the more comprehensive your care will be. I mean, if you're not comfortable telling this person who you're sleeping with, what you're smoking, or how often you have diarrhea, you're not really getting your money's worth.

So it's not unreasonable to have some preferences when it comes to who that person is. Would you be more comfortable seeing someone of your same gender? Your same sexual orientation? Someone who shares your racial or ethnic identity? Or shares your religious beliefs? Really take a moment to think about the kind of medical setting that would make you feel most comfortable. You are allowed to be picky when it comes to your personal health and safety, even though this, unfortunately, can make finding care that you can afford and access even harder.

Finally, don't downplay the importance of a good vibe. When I'm choosing a provider, vibe is as important as credentials. You never want to feel rushed, judged, or patronized—especially not when your ass is hanging out the back of a hospital gown.

My hope is that you're able to use the lessons in the previous chapters to find authoritative experts to make up your care team who check off the following boxes:

- They have the appropriate credentials, certifications, or affiliations associated with a high degree of experience in the specific topic you're seeing them about.

- They aren't overly interested in selling you something that only they have access to.

- They provide recommendations and treatments that are evidence-based, and you're able to verify that evidence using the methods you learned in this book.

- They treat you with respect and dignity, at an absolute minimum.

Use that checklist the next time you need a gynecologist, a nutritionist, a physical therapist, a psychiatrist, a primary care provider, or something else.

Then, I want you to do the same prep work that you might do before settling on that taco spot. Look to see if they have a website, reviews, or pictures of the location that might help you get a sense of the practice. Call ahead to try to get as much information as you can about pricing. (Do they take your insurance? Can they tell you what you'll actually owe after the first visit? If you might need to get any tests or bloodwork done, is that done on-site or would you need to go somewhere else?) And if you think you'd have a better experience and feel more comfortable with someone by your side, bring that person with you.

I know this all sounds like a lot of work, but I promise it's worth it to do this preparation from the comfort of your couch, rather than trying to get answers when you're already flustered and late for work after your appointment.

HOW TO ACTUALLY FIND A PROVIDER

TRY SEARCHING ON ZOCDOC OR SHARECARE: While their usefulness really varies depending on where you live, both of these websites let you filter your search by location, insurance provider, availability, and patient reviews. I'm personally a huge fan of Zocdoc because it lets you make an appointment and fill out your paperwork online, plus they send you helpful notifications—like when it's somehow been a year already since your last dentist appointment. Just make sure to call the provider directly and confirm that they take your insurance, even if the site says they do. Trust me on this one—it takes five minutes and could save you a whole lot of hassle and money.

VISIT YOUR INSURANCE COMPANY'S WEBSITE: If you're insured, you should be able to find a database of in-network providers on your insurance company's website. I've found these are usually pretty bare-bones when it comes to providing things like bios, photos, and patient reviews, so my suggestion would be to copy and paste a provider's name into a search engine to find out more about them that way. It's time-consuming, but at least you know they're already in-network.

TRY A TELEMEDICINE APP LIKE TELADOC OR MDLIVE: These services might be covered under your insurance policy, so they're worth checking out if it's typically hard for you to get to a doctor's office based on your schedule/location/life. While I wouldn't suggest telemedicine as your primary care provider, it's a really helpful tool for those times when you're dealing with something run-of-the-mill like a sinus infection or UTI and you can't or don't want to get to a doctor's office. Even if you don't have health insurance, you can typically pay per visit with a credit card, the same way you would at a walk-in urgent care center.

FOR A MENTAL HEALTH PROVIDER, TRY THE FOLLOWING WEBSITES: Psychology Today, Therapy for Black Girls, and SAMHSA (Substance Abuse and Mental Health Services Administration) are all great resources for finding licensed mental health providers in your area.

Know that not having insurance doesn't mean you don't deserve the same level of care.

More than 26 million people in the United States did not have health insurance at all during 2019, according to data from the U.S. Census Bureau.[60] A significant chunk of that data was collected in March 2020, at the very beginning of the COVID-19 pandemic, so it's worth considering how that affected response rates at the time, as well as how different those numbers might be for 2020 coverage. For instance, 55.4 percent of people in 2019 reported getting their health insurance through their employer, and I know far too many people who lost their jobs in 2020.

We know that insurance status is a strong determining factor when it comes to taking care of your health—whether it's getting your routine health screenings or staying on lifesaving medications. And it's not hard to see why: Medical care is expensive as hell, even with insurance. And when you're making a decision about what to spend your money on, it's really hard to make the case for something as intangible as your health. That medical bill is tangible—you can see it and feel it. Those test results, on the other hand, are much harder to size up. Will it be worth the money to get the all clear? Will pushing it off for 6 or 12 more months make a difference? Will you end up with news that you and your bank account just aren't ready to deal with?

One of my biggest gripes is one-size-fits-all health information and advice—whether it's in magazine articles, online, or in daytime talk show segments—that make the assumption that everyone is in the same boat. That everyone has health insurance, not to mention the time and resources to pop in for a physical, a colonoscopy, bloodwork, genetic testing, whatever. For at least 26 million people, it's not that simple, and it can be demoralizing to hear that it is.

So I am not going to sit here and tell you that—insured or not—you need to find a way to prioritize your health. I know it's not that simple. Instead, I'm going to tell you that I'm sorry that the health information out there is overwhelmingly dismissive and ignorant of your experience and your circumstances. That sucks. We have to stop pretending that health care is one-size-fits-all.

> *We have to stop pretending that health care is one-size-fits-all.*

My hunch is that this approach persists because it is so much harder to speak to a wider range of people and experiences when you're talking about health. Trust me—it's taken me far longer than I expected to write this chapter. And as I sat here thinking *this is too hard, I don't know if I can do this,* I realized how illustrative that is of the experience that more than 26 million people in this country deal with every day. It's hard and it's complicated and it's not uncommon to become so overwhelmed and defeated that you put it off or give up entirely. I get it. But I also want you to know that just because your experience and circumstances are not centered in mainstream health media, that doesn't mean that you are not deserving of accessible, empathetic, evidence-based care. It doesn't mean you don't have options outside of the emergency department.

This is by no means an exhaustive list of resources for anyone who is uninsured or underinsured, but my hope is that it shows you that options are out there for you. If you can, try not to skip it.

○ **Find a community health center:** Health centers provide primary care and other important health care services like mental health and substance use support on a sliding scale, depending on your income and family size. If you're uninsured or underinsured, go to Findahealthcenter.HRSA.gov to find a health center near you.

○ **Look to your state health department:** If you're looking for something specific—vaccinations, family planning services, mammograms, STD testing—I suggest you start by searching for your state's health department website. Once you find the site for your state, poke around a bit in the subject area you're interested in. You can expect to see information on federally funded programs as well as low- or no-cost services for uninsured or low-income individuals. Fair warning: It's not as easy as it should be to find this information. If you're having trouble, look for a Contact Us page and try to get someone on the phone who can help you get to what you're looking for.

○ **Check with Planned Parenthood:** If you need birth control, STD and HIV testing, pelvic exams, or pregnancy and abortion services, Planned Parenthood is often a convenient and affordable resource. Depending on the center, you can also go there for general health screenings, cancer screenings, flu shots, smoking cessation, hormone therapy, and more. Services are typically provided on a sliding scale, but I would suggest calling before you go to find out what you can expect to pay for the services you need.

○ **See if you qualify for Medicaid:** This is unfortunately another process that is unnecessarily difficult to navigate, but it's worth looking into if you could benefit from free or low-cost health coverage. Medicaid eligibility varies by state, but it's generally based on income, pregnancy, disability, and the number of people in your household. Healthcare.gov will be your starting point to determine eligibility; from there, you'll likely be directed to resources specific to your state and circumstances.

○ **Save on prescription medications with a little research:** Raise your hand if you've ever gotten sticker shock at the pharmacy counter but you were too flustered/embarrassed/confused to do anything but pay whatever they're asking. Same. But let's not do that anymore. The next time you get a prescription from your doctor, take an hour to do some comparison shopping. For starters, you can ask for the generic option rather than the name brand if there's one available. Generics aren't any less effective. If there's no generic option, Google the name brand of the medication to see if the company offers any coupons on its website—many of them do. You can also search online for prescription discount services, like GoodRx or Optum Perks. These sites show you what price you can expect to pay for the exact same medication depending on the pharmacy and coupon you use. And you can take advantage of these discounts whether you have insurance or not.

Ask so many questions, and know that you are deserving of answers.

If you take away one thing from this book, I sure hope you remember the importance—not to mention the power—of asking questions. Because I promise you aren't the only one who has whatever question you feel too silly or uninformed to ask.

"People are not alone in their confusion," Lisa Fitzpatrick, MD, founder of Grapevine Health, tells me. "People feel embarrassed and ashamed to ask these questions because they feel like they should know."

Fitzpatrick is a CDC-trained epidemiologist and board-certified infectious disease physician. Most of us would be a little intimidated to have a conversation with a medical expert like that, but that's the exact opposite vibe you get when speaking with Fitzpatrick. Maybe that's because she spends so much of her time speaking directly to the public—not in an exam room or onstage at a TED Talk (though she's also done that), but on the streets of their communities. Since 2013, Fitzpatrick has been filming a YouTube series called Dr. Lisa On The Street, where she quite literally meets patients where they are to help demystify medical topics—from diabetes to telehealth to COVID-19.

I asked Fitzpatrick what advice she finds herself giving over and over again to people who are struggling to either find care or act on that care.

"I think the biggest repeat piece of advice I'm giving people is you need to get all your questions answered until you're satisfied," Fitzpatrick tells me. "And if they say something you don't understand, interrupt them, because people don't feel like they have the authority to do that."

Ask questions. Ask all your questions. Ask the obvious questions. Ask the same questions to multiple people. Ask if you're understanding something correctly. Ask why—a lot. Ask for a minute to make sure that you've asked all your questions. And if you have a hard time asking questions of all those people in white coats, ask yourself why that is.

> *Ask questions. Ask all your questions. Ask the obvious questions. Ask the same questions to multiple people.*

I became a better health editor by asking a shit ton of questions to a shit ton of experts. And I became a little bit more comfortable with my body by doing the same thing. The unfortunate reality is that most health care providers have very little time to spend with each patient, so it's natural to feel rushed—like you're holding them up. But remember: You are a paying customer here. And this isn't some low-stakes thing like wanting to ask for more hot sauce but also not wanting to bother your busy server. This is your body, your health. Ask your questions, and remember that you are deserving of answers.

Notice here that I didn't say "demand answers," because the truth is that sometimes even the brightest minds in medicine will not have an answer for you. And as frustrating as that can be, it's not as frustrating as someone pulling an answer out of their ass just to appease you. After interviewing a lot of experts about a lot of subjects, I can tell you that I personally don't want to see a provider who has all the answers. I want someone who will tell me when they don't have an answer and will promise me that they're going to try to help me anyway.

There is a difference between demanding an answer and knowing that you are *deserving of* answers. Demanding an answer looks like not being willing to leave a doctor's office without a prescription—regardless of whether or not there's any evidence to suggest it'll help you. Not only is this frustrating for everyone involved, but it's also not likely to get you any closer to feeling better.

Being deserving of answers looks like not being afraid to ask your doctor to explain something in more detail. It looks like standing your ground when they tell you "that can't be right" when you explain to them what you're experiencing. It looks like getting a second opinion when they recommend something costly and complicated without being able to explain to you why it's the best course of treatment for you. It means reminding yourself that you're not being annoying or irrational for having a whole lot of questions about what's going on in your body.

Know that you are not a burden.

I want to leave you with a story about my grandma, a person I miss deeply every day. Her name was Dorothy, but she was Grandma Dottie to all of our closest friends. I was lucky enough to live under the same roof as my grandma from as early as I can remember until I was 14, when she passed away. I'm told often that I have her nose. I also have her anxiety and her nervous stomach, neither of which are particularly lovely things to inherit, but I love what it means: that I came from her, that parts of my genetic makeup are just like hers.

"I don't want to be a burden," my grandma would say to any one of us, practically once a day.

She said it in a sort of singsong way, often as she was leaving a room so as not to give the person on the receiving end a chance to say she was being ridiculous, that she wasn't a burden. She said it so often that my family and I still recite it sometimes as a joke, when we feel like we're being difficult but secretly know that we're not.

See, my grandma was not a burden. She played an enormous role in raising me, the youngest of three girls who often needed a babysitter or a playmate while my older sisters were shuttled off to school, sleepovers, and extracurricular activities. She entertained us, educated us, loved us, bought us the very best the Home Shopping Network had to offer. She was a crucial part of our family, of our household. But she often thought she was being burdensome—by needing help, having an opinion, or just generally existing.

I can imagine that she felt like a burden living with us all those years, even though the reality was that she provided far more than she ever asked for in return. And I can imagine that she felt like a burden when she needed to see a doctor or go to the pharmacy, since she didn't drive and she did have a handful of health issues. I'm sure she felt like a burden when she fell once and broke both of her wrists, which led to a few months in which my mom helped her perform pretty much every task you can imagine . . . and a few you'd rather not.

But no one in my family would have ever characterized her that way. You aren't a burden for needing help with your basic needs.

So why do so many of us feel like a burden anytime we have a question or concern or need regarding our health? We feel like we're taking up the doctor's time. We're asking too many questions. We should know what they're talking about, what that big word means, and in what order to take those four medications they just rattled off. We feel too awkward and uncomfortable to speak our minds or ask for clarification. We straight up avoid getting medical attention unless we're basically on fire, for fear of a false alarm. *It's probably nothing,* we tell ourselves—because we don't want to be a burden.

If you can relate to that feeling, I want to tell you the same thing I mumbled after Grandma Dottie each time she said her peace and turned to walk away; the same thing I wish I could tell her today. You are not a burden.

- You are not a burden for not already magically knowing exactly how to take care of your health.

- You are not a burden for texting your best friend in the middle of the night to ask if you're dying.

- You are not a burden for asking a health care provider to explain something in a way you'll actually understand.

- And you are certainly not a burden for needing assistance—physical, emotional, financial, or otherwise—to better care for yourself, to live.

The next time you feel embarrassed, uninformed, needy, or broken because of a health concern, I hope you won't let that feeling linger in the air, as if your inner voice dropped it there and then walked away before you could contradict it.

Trust me, you are not a burden.

ACKNOWLEDGMENTS

First and foremost, thank you to everyone who picked up this book—for yourself or someone else. I am so grateful (and, frankly, blown away) that people read and share my work.

A huge thank you to my agent Leila Campoli for shepherding this book into existence while somehow keeping my stress levels in check. You made this writer an author. I am incredibly grateful for my brilliant editor, Shannon Connors Fabricant, I couldn't have asked for a more perfect partner in this journey. Your insightful guidance and genuine enthusiasm for this book is a true gift. Susan Van Horn, thank you for the beautiful cover and interior designs that bring this book to life.

Thank you to all of the amazing writers and editors who shaped my work over the years: Carolyn Kylstra, Zahra Barnes, Anna Borges, Sarah Jacoby, Robin Hilmantel, Caroline Kee, Ben Smith, Kate White, John Searles, Bethany Heitman, Jessica Knoll, Andrea Bartz, and so many more. A very special thank you to Sally Tamarkin, my dear friend, fact-checker, and sensitivity reader—this book (and basically all of my work) is better because of your discerning eye and thoughtful feedback.

Sincerest thank you to all of the experts who lent their time and insights to this book . . . in a pandemic, no less. I am awestruck by each one of you, and I still can't believe I get to talk to you and call it work. Jen Gunter, I truly teared up when reading your incredible foreword. Thank you for sharing so many kind and wise words over the years.

Thank you to the most supportive and inspiring group of friends on this planet. Kristen, I can't remember a time in my life when you weren't there for me, and I never want to. Kate, thank you for being a part of almost every story in here—I can't begin to tell you how thankful I am for our friendship. Mel, I am so lucky to have you—and your medical expertise—in my life. Lauren, thank you for always bringing me home, literally and figuratively.

Kenny, thank you for being the best emergency contact a girl could ask for. To Andrew, Albert, Kevin, Amanda, Kaysee, my Cru girls, and plenty more, thank you for the much-needed support, laughs, drinks, and debriefs that kept me going while I tapped away at this.

And to my big, beautiful, blended family, thank you for showing me time and again that family is always there. To my siblings: Amy, Lindsay, Tori, Taylor, Brian, Cody, how did I get so lucky to get all of you for life? To Linda and Peter, thank you for loving me like a daughter. To Brien and Kinsley, you'll blow us all away.

To my Mom and Dad, thank you for always reminding me that I am loved, supported, and capable of doing hard things. I am so deeply thankful to have you in my corner. This book is for you.

NOTES

1 American Psychiatric Association, *Diagnostic and Statistical Manual of Mental Disorders: DSM-5* (Arlington, VA: American Psychiatric Association, 2013).

2 American Psychiatric Association, *Diagnostic and Statistical Manual of Mental Disorders: DSM-5* (Arlington, VA: American Psychiatric Association, 2013).

3 "Move to Be Well: The Global Economy of Physical Activity," Global Wellness Institute, October 2019, https://globalwellnessinstitute.org/wp-content/uploads/2019/10/2019-Physical-Activity-Economy-FINAL-NEW-101019.pdf.

4 John Weinman, Gibran Yusuf et al., "How accurate is patients' anatomical knowledge: a cross-sectional, questionnaire study of six patient groups and a general public sample," *BMC Family Practice* 10, 43 (2009), https://doi.org/10.1186/1471-2296-10-43.

5 Victoria Waldersee, "Half of Brits don't know where the vagina is—and it's not just the men," YouGov, March 8, 2019, https://yougov.co.uk/topics/health/articles-reports/2019/03/08/half-brits-dont-know-where-vagina-and-its-not-just.

6 "How Millennials approach health care," HealthPocket, December 20, 2019, https://www.healthpocket.com/healthcare-research/surveys/how-millennials-approach-health-insurance#.X2-ewtNKjjA.

7 "Results from the School Health Policies and Practices Study," Centers for Disease Control and Prevention, 2016, Table 1.1, https://www.cdc.gov/healthyyouth/data/shpps/pdf/shpps-results_2016.pdf#page=20.

8 "School Health Profiles: 2018, Characteristics of Health Programs Among Secondary Schools," Centers for Disease Control and Prevention, 2019, https://www.cdc.gov/healthyyouth/data/profiles/pdf/2018/CDC-Profiles-2018.pdf.

9 "School Enrollment in the United States: October 2018—Detailed Tables," United States Census Bureau, Table 1, Last revised December 3, 2019, https://www.census.gov/data/tables/2018/demo/school-enrollment/2018-cps.html.

10 "School Health Profiles: 2018, Characteristics of Health Programs Among Secondary Schools," Centers for Disease Control and Prevention, 2019, https://www.cdc.gov/healthyyouth/data/profiles/pdf/2018/CDC-Profiles-2018.pdf.

11 Selden, Catherine R.; Zorn, Marcia; Ratzan, Scott; Parker, Ruth M., compilers. Health literacy [bibliography online]. Bethesda (MD): National Library of Medicine; 2000 Feb. (Current bibliographies in medicine; no. 2000-1). 479 citations from January 1989 through December 1999. Available from: https://www.nlm.nih.gov/archive/20061214/pubs/cbm/hliteracy.html.

12 U.S. Department of Health and Human Services, Office of Disease Prevention and Health Promotion. (2010). National Action Plan to Improve Health Literacy. Washington, DC: Author. https://health.gov/sites/default/files/2019-09/Health_Literacy_Action_Plan.pdf.

13 "Media Literacy Defined," National Association for Media Literacy Education, accessed September 26, 2020, https://namle.net/publications/media-literacy-defined/.

14 J. E. R. Staddon et al., "Operant Conditioning," *Annual Review of Psychology*, 54 (February 2003): https://doi.org/10.1146/annurev.psych.54.101601.145124.

15 "Everything You Need to Know About the Google Medic Update," Wpromote, September 13, 2018, https://www.wpromote.com/blog/seo/everything-need-know-google-medic-update.

16 Richard S. Bradbury et al., "A Second Case of Human Conjunctival Infestation with Thelazia gulosa and a Review of T. gulosa in North America," *Clinical Infectious Diseases* 70, no. 3 (February 2020): 518–520, https://doi.org/10.1093/cid/ciz469.

17 Maria Naranjo et al., "Sudden Death of a Young Adult Associated with *Bacillus cereus* Food Poisoning," *Journal of Clinical Microbiology* 49, no. 12 (December 2011): 4379–4381, https://doi.org/10.1128/JCM.05129-11.

18 James Felton, "A student died in his sleep after eating 5-day-old pasta that had been left out," Business Insider, January 29, 2019, https://www.businessinsider.com/student-died-in-his-sleep-after-eating-5-day-old-pasta-that-had-been-left-out-2019-1.

19 Chubbyemu, "A Student Ate 5 Day Old Pasta For Lunch. This Is How His Liver Shut Down," YouTube, January 21, 2019, https://www.youtube.com/watch?v=5ujTYLV2Qo4.

20 Saskia Verkaik et al., "The treatment of premenstrual syndrome with preparations of *Vitex agnus castus*: a systematic review and meta-analysis," *American Journal of Obstetrics and Gynecology* 217, no. 2 (August 2017): 150–166, https://doi.org/10.1016/j.ajog.2017.02.028.

21 Birgit M. Dietz et al., "Botanicals and Their Bioactive Phytochemicals for Women's Health," *Pharmacological Reviews* 68, no. 4 (October 2016): 1026–1073, https://doi.org/10.1124/pr.115.010843.

22 "About Chronic Diseases," National Center for Chronic Disease Prevention and Health Promotion, Centers for Disease Control, last reviewed October 23, 2019, https://www.cdc.gov/chronicdisease/about/index.htm.

23 Sheldon Cohen et al., "Psychological stress and susceptibility to the common cold," *New England Journal of Medicine* 325, no. 9 (September 1991): 606–612, https://doi.org/10.1056/NEJM199108293250903.

24 Ulrik Deding et al., "Perceived stress as a risk factor for peptic ulcers: a register-based cohort study," *BMC Gastroenterology* 16, no. 140 (November 2016), https://doi.org/10.1186/s12876-016-0554-9.

25 "Stress Can Increase Your Risk for Heart Disease," Health Encyclopedia, University of Rochester Medical Center, accessed September 26, 2020, https://www.urmc.rochester.edu/encyclopedia/content.aspx?ContentTypeID=1&ContentID=2171.

26 American Heart Association News, "Stress May Increase Type 2 Diabetes Risk in Women," American Heart Association, November 6, 2018, https://www.heart.org/en/news/2018/11/06/stress-may-increase-type-2-diabetes-risk-in-women.

27 Hong-Yan Qin et al., "Impact of psychological stress on irritable bowel syndrome," World Journal of Gastroenterology 20, no. 39 (October 2014): 14126–14131, https://doi.org/10.3748/wjg.v20.i39.14126.

28 J. E. Mawdsley and D. S. Rampton, "Psychological stress in IBD: new insights into pathogenic and therapeutic implications," Gut 54, no. 10 (October 2005): 1481–1491, https://doi.org/10.1136/gut.2005.064261.

29 Nasim Maleki, Lino Becerra, and David Borsook, "Migraine: Maladaptive Brain Responses to Stress," Headache 52, no. 2 (October 2012): 102–106, https://doi.org/10.1111/j.1526-4610.2012.02241.x.

30 David C. Mohr et al., "Association between stressful life events and exacerbation in multiple sclerosis: a meta-analysis," BMJ 328, no. 731 (March 2004), https://doi.org/10.1136/bmj.38041.724421.55.

31 Arline T. Geronimus et al., "'Weathering' and Age Patterns of Allostatic Load Scores Among Blacks and Whites in the United States,'" American Journal of Public Health 96, no. 5 (May 2006): 826–833, https://doi.org/10.2105/AJPH.2004.060749.

32 U.S. Cancer Statistics Working Group, U.S. Cancer Statistics Data Visualizations Tool, based on 2019 submission data (1999–2017): U.S. Department of Health and Human Services, Centers for Disease Control and Prevention and National Cancer Institute; released in June 2020, https://gis.cdc.gov/Cancer/USCS/DataViz.html.

33 "Disease Burden of Influenza," Influenza (Flu), Centers for Disease Control and Prevention, last reviewed October 5, 2020, https://www.cdc.gov/flu/about/burden/index.html.

34 "How CDC Estimates Burden," Influenza (Flu), Centers for Disease Control and Prevention, last reviewed November 22, 2019, https://www.cdc.gov/flu/about/burden/how-cdc-estimates.htm.

35 Press Association, "Up to 25 cups of coffee a day safe for heart health, study finds," The Guardian, June 2, 2019, https://www.theguardian.com/food/2019/jun/02/up-to-25-cups-of-coffee-a-day-safe-for-heart-health-study-finds.

36 Bob Fredericks, "Cabbage could help fight COVID-19, study finds," New York Post, July 20, 2020, https://nypost.com/2020/07/20/foods-containing-cabbage-could-help-fight-coronavirus/.

37 Tony Merevick, "Drinking Champagne Is Good for Your Brain and Prevents Memory Loss," Thrillist, November 9, 2015, https://www.thrillist.com/news/nation/drinking-champagne-is-good-for-your-brain-and-prevents-memory-loss.

38 Giulia Corona et al., "Phenolic Acid Intake, Delivered Via Moderate Champagne Wine Consumption, Improves Spatial Working Memory Via the Modulation of Hippocampal and Cortical Protein Expression/Activation," Antioxidants & Redox Signaling 19, no. 14 (October 2013), https://doi.org/10.1089/ars.2012.5142.

39 Table A7.1, Appendix 7, 2015–2020 Dietary Guidelines for Americans, 8th Edition, December 2015, https://health.gov/our-work/food-nutrition/2015-2020-dietary-guidelines/guidelines/appendix-7/.

40 Carolyn Todd, "Why Some Bars Make You Crampy, Farty, and Bloated," *SELF*, September 24, 2019, https://www.self.com/story/protein-fiber-bars-gas-bloating-cramps.

41 Practice Committee of the American Society for Reproductive Medicine, "Combined hormonal contraception and the risk of venous thromboembolism: a guideline," *Fertility and Sterility* 107, no. 1 (January 2017): 43–51, https://doi.org/10.1016/j.fertnstert.2016.09.027.

42 Yana Vinogradova et al., "Use of combined oral contraceptives and risk of venous thromboembolism: nested case-control studies using the QResearch and CPRD databases," *BMJ* 350 (May 2015), https://doi.org/10.1136/bmj.h2135.

43 Elizabeth Narins, "Why Are Women Dying From Taking the Pill?" *Cosmopolitan*, May 28, 2015, https://www.cosmopolitan.com/health-fitness/advice/a41060/why-people-are-dying-from-the-pill/.

44 Steven Tenny and Ibrahim Abdelgawad, "Statistical Significance," StatPearls, July 10, 2020, https://www.ncbi.nlm.nih.gov/books/NBK459346/.

45 Anna Medaris Miller, "Experts warn birth-control pills could increase the risk of 'deadly blood clots' in coronavirus patients," Insider, July 29, 2020, https://www.insider.com/birth-control-may-lead-to-blood-clots-in-coronavirus-patients-2020-7.

46 Daniel I. Spratt and Rachel J. Buchsbaum, "COVID-19 and Hypercoagulability: Potential Impact on Management with Oral Contraceptives, Estrogen Therapy, and Pregnancy," *Endocrinology* (July 2020), https://doi.org/10.1056/NEJM199108293250903.

47 Antiperspirants/Deodorants and Breast Cancer, National Cancer Institute, reviewed August 9, 2016, https://www.cancer.gov/about-cancer/causes-prevention/risk/myths/antiperspirants-fact-sheet.

48 "Probiotics: What You Need to Know," National Center for Complementary and Integrative Heath, last updated August 2019, https://www.nccih.nih.gov/health/probiotics-what-you-need-to-know.

49 "The Facts on Tampons and How to Use Them Safely," FDA, last reviewed September 12, 2018, https://www.fda.gov/consumers/consumer-updates/facts-tampons-and-how-use-them-safely.

50 "Dioxins and their effects on human health," World Health Organization, October 4, 2016, https://www.who.int/en/news-room/fact-sheets/detail/dioxins-and-their-effects-on-human-health.

51 Christopher Kirkpatrick, "Acute Macular Neuroretinopathy (AMN)" EyeRounds.org, last updated September 30, 2016, https://eyerounds.org/atlas/pages/Acute-macular-neuroretinopathy/index.htm.

52 Kavita V. Bhavsar et al., "Acute macular neuroretinopathy: A comprehensive review of the literature," *Survey of Ophthalmology* 61, no. 5 (September 2016): 538–565, https://doi.org/10.1016/j.survophthal.2016.03.003.

53 Carmen Arriola et al., "Influenza Vaccination Modifies Disease Severity Among Community-dwelling Adults Hospitalized With Influenza," *Clinical Infectious Diseases* 65, no. 8 (October 2017): 1289–1297, https://doi.org/10.1093/cid/cix468.

54 "Cancer Prevention & Early Detection Facts & Figures 2019–2020," American Cancer Society, 2019, https://www.cancer.org/content/dam/cancer-org/research/cancer-facts-and-statistics/cancer-prevention-and-early-detection-facts-and-figures/cancer-prevention-and-early-detection-facts-and-figures-2019-2020.pdf.

55 "Survival Rates for Cervical Cancer," American Cancer Society, last revised January 3, 2020, https://www.cancer.org/cancer/cervical-cancer/detection-diagnosis-staging/survival.html.

56 "Cancer Prevention & Early Detection Facts & Figures 2019–2020," American Cancer Society, 2019, https://www.cancer.org/content/dam/cancer-org/research/cancer-facts-and-statistics/cancer-prevention-and-early-detection-facts-and-figures/cancer-prevention-and-early-detection-facts-and-figures-2019-2020.pdf.

57 "What Can I Do to Reduce My Risk?" Colorectal (Colon) Cancer, Centers for Disease Control and Prevention, last reviewed February 10, 2020, https://www.cdc.gov/cancer/colorectal/basic_info/prevention.htm.

58 "Cancer Prevention & Early Detection Facts & Figures 2019–2020," American Cancer Society, 2019, https://www.cancer.org/content/dam/cancer-org/research/cancer-facts-and-statistics/cancer-prevention-and-early-detection-facts-and-figures/cancer-prevention-and-early-detection-facts-and-figures-2019-2020.pdf.

59 "Facts About Hypertension," High Blood Pressure, Centers for Disease Control and Prevention, last reviewed September 8, 2020, https://www.cdc.gov/bloodpressure/facts.htm.

60 Katherine Keisler-Starkey and Lisa N. Bunch, "Health Insurance Coverage in the United States: 2019," U.S. Census Bureau, Issued September 2020, https://www.census.gov/content/dam/Census/library/publications/2020/demo/p60-271.pdf.

INDEX

Health concerns. *See also* Women's
    health
    asking questions, 38, 192–196
    "burdens," 194–196
    demystifying, 192–193
    health anxiety and, 5–23, 49–65,
        96–102
    sources for checking, 171–174
Health department, 191
Health education
    accessing, 84
    failure of, 27–34
    health literacy and, 38–45
    media literacy and, 18, 46–48
    scholarly articles, 174–176
    sex education, 31–38
    standards for, 33–36
    understanding, 2, 27–36
Health equity, 181
Health hack, 182–184
Health headlines
    absolute risk, 136–137
    abundance of, 20–21, 62–64,
        77–80, 94, 113–115
    causation and, 132–136
    coronavirus and, 111–114, 132–
        133, 141–142
    correlation and, 132–136
    decoding, 20–21, 113–145

expertise and, 115–145
fact-checking, 121–123, 126–127,
    143–145
health literacy and, 18–21
health reporting and, 10–13
media outlets and, 119–145
pandemic and, 111–114, 132–
    133, 141–142
primary sources, 123–126
qualifications and, 115–145
relative risk, 136–137
research and, 127–135, 138–139,
    142
reviews of, 143–144
risks and, 136–138, 141–142
scholarly articles, 174–176
secondary sources, 123–126
significant risk, 139
signs/symptoms articles, 58–66
sources of, 47, 115–145
studies and, 127–134, 138–139
Health insurance
    access to, 181
    affording, 181
    concerns about, 54, 57
    deductibles, 180
    health care crisis, 179–181
    health equity, 181
    health resources, 190–192

National Institute of Diabetes and Digestive and Kidney Diseases, 172

National Institute of Mental Health, 172

National Institutes of Health (NIH), 47, 121

National Library of Medicine, 172

National Sleep Foundation, 172

Natural products, 71–72, 83, 147, 152–156

New York Times, 144

"Normal," 22–23, 27

NYU Langone, 161, 173

O

Obsessive-compulsive disorder (OCD), 15–17, 96, 106

Operant conditioning, 52–54

Optum Perks, 192

P

Pandemic
    causation and, 132–133
    concerns about, 56
    flu season and, 124–126
    headlines and, 111–114, 132–133, 141–142
    health insurance and, 189
    rashes and, 166–167
    reporting on, 19, 40, 46

Panic attacks, 5–6, 20, 103–109

Panic disorder, 15

Pap smears, 2, 5–6, 39–40, 164–165, 171, 183–184

Physical exams, 12–13, 74, 184

Planned Parenthood, 122, 172, 191

PMS symptoms, 67–69

Pregnancy, 12, 32, 49–50, 137–138, 191

Prescription medications, 172, 179–180, 191–192. *See also* Medications

Preventive care, 172, 182–184, 189–191

Prognosis, 43, 107

Psychology Today, 188

PubMed, 67, 176

Q

Qualifications
    accredited degrees, 117–118
    biases, 133–134, 140–141
    certifications, 117–118
    conflicts of interest, 120–121, 140–141
    experience, 117–121
    finding experts, 170–174
    health headlines and, 115–145
    health sources and, 117–145, 171–174
    media outlets and, 119–145